R
860
M66
1995

2-12-04

04-0366

Health and Safety Guidelines for the Laboratory

	DATE DUE		

MILLER-MOTTE TECHNICAL
COLLEGE LIBRARY

D1511695

R
860
M66
1995

Health and Safety Guidelines for the Laboratory

Lynn Montgomery, CPM, CT, HT(ASCP)

Baton Rouge, Louisiana

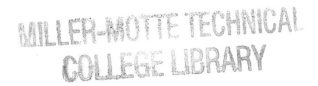
MILLER-MOTTE TECHNICAL
COLLEGE LIBRARY

Library of Congress Cataloging-in-Publication Data

Montgomery, Lynn.
Health and safety guidelines for the laboratory/Lynn Montgomery.
p. cm.
Includes bibliographical references.
ISBN 0-89189-382-2
1. Medical Laboratories—Safety Measures—Standards—United States. I. Title.
[DNLM: 1. Laboratories—standards—United States— legislation.
2. Occupational Exposure—standards—United States—legislation.
3. Occupational Health—United States—legislation.   WA 33 AA1 M7h
1994]
R860.M66   1994
610'.724—dc20
DNLM/DLC   94-8501
for Library of Congress CIP

Copyright© 1995 by The American Society of Clinical Pathologists.
All rights reserved. No part of this publication may be reproduced, stored in a retrieval system, or transmitted in any form or by any means, electronic, mechanical, photocopying, recording, or otherwise, without the prior written permission of the publisher.

Printed in the United States of America.

99 98 97 96 95   5 4 3 2 1

Table of Contents

Dedication

To the one who understood and believed in the "Divine Miss M." For this, I am forever changed.

Preface

To compile a text that would detail each of the Occupational Safety and Health Administration (OSHA) regulations that now make an impact on our laboratories would be a monumental if not impossible task. Because of the ever-increasing demands on laboratory personnel and their need for concise, readily accessible information, this manual provides clearly defined basic guidelines and information to assist laboratorians in preparing health and safety programs. The manual will not only aid in developing programs that will be in compliance with the OSHA standards but also serve as a comprehensive and highly usable reference for everyday laboratory needs.

The text primarily deals with the Hazard Communication Standard (the Right-to-Know Law), the Formaldehyde Standard, the Occupational Exposures to Hazardous Chemicals in Laboratories Standard (frequently called the Laboratory Standard and containing the Chemical Hygiene Plan), and the Bloodborne Pathogen Standard. Additional information is included regarding regulatory agencies, successful compliance, latex sensitivity, and handling radiological materials. Also included is information on laboratory waste management and guidelines for prevention of transmission of tuberculosis in health care facilities. A section for laboratory self-evaluation on compliance with these standards is also included, along with an extensive glossary and resource information.

This text describes the essentials of the standards, interpreting the basic requirements for compliance and the scope and terminology of the laws. The basic guidelines for regulatory compliance are presented along with examples and suggestions. The focus of this text is the nature of the requirements and the steps necessary for implementation. The text does not, however, attempt to explain all aspects of the laws in detail, but presents the general structure of the documents. It is written by a technologist primarily for technologists, and does not represent a legal interpretation of the law in any manner. When questions regarding compliance arise, it is always best to refer to the standard as printed in the *Federal Register*. Every laboratory should have a complete copy of each standard. Compliance requirements may vary from state to state or even city to city depending on local ordinances that may supersede the OSHA regulations. There may exist an overlap between federal and state regulations, and between agencies at any of these levels. When establishing any program for regulatory standard compliance, local and state regulations should be considered by each laboratory on an individual basis.

OSHA standards are written with considerable flexibility, recognizing the various differences in laboratories; often individual interpretation of these standards can cause considerable misunderstanding. Too often, the laboratory becomes so concerned with compliance that the initial intent of these regulations and guidelines becomes lost in an effort to "pass inspection." Frequently, blanket mandates are passed down through sections of the laboratory, which may or may not be necessary or required by the standards. Some administrators get so bogged down in minute details of the standards that they completely lose sight of the original objective of the legislation and produce a program that is so detailed and cumbersome that it loses its effectiveness. Understand the original intent of these standards, which is to provide a safer workplace, and resist the urge to overreact to compliance mandates. An important aspect of compliance is that OSHA requires each laboratory to develop its own individual programs. The standards are written in a clearly stated outline form with definitions of terminology and numerous examples. Do not hesitate to call OSHA for assistance with questions regarding these regulations. The information is free and you will save yourself considerable time and confusion. For this purpose, an extensive list of phone numbers is provided at the end of this manual.

It is important that the reader understand that while the information contained in this manual is as up-to-date as possible, the constantly changing nature of government regulations will render some of this material obsolete by the time the final version of these regulations is issued. Specifically, new standards addressing ergonomics and the prevention of transmission of tuberculosis in health care facilities are being finalized by OSHA as this manual goes to press. The reader must be alert to this constantly changing regulatory environment.

Laboratory medicine and our laboratories have undergone a tremendous evolution in the past 10 years. We are moving into the 21st century with a new sense of environmental awareness and increased understanding of our chemical and biological exposures. We have moved from frequently hazardous, polluted laboratories into safer, healthier workplaces. I am confident that the best is yet to come!

Lynn Montgomery, BS, CPM, CT/HT(ASCP)
Baton Rouge, Louisiana

Acknowledgments

There are numerous people whom I would like to thank for their encouragement and faith in the completion of this book, too numerous, in fact, to list here. I have surely been blessed with wonderful colleagues and kind friends who have supported this publication. I sincerely thank them all. I would particularly like to thank Cheryl Crowder, Pamela Stratton, and Rosemary Klein, Louisiana State University School of Veterinary Medicine, Baton Rouge; Joy Reuter; Rena Krol, Gulf Coast Research Laboratories, Ocean Springs, Mississippi; Mary Anne Tourres, East Jefferson Hospital, Metairie, Louisiana; Glenda Hood, Parkland Hospital, Dallas, Texas; and Beena Rao, ASCP Editor.

Chapter 1

Introduction to Regulatory Standards

1.1 INTRODUCTION TO OSHA AND OTHER REGULATORY AGENCIES

When most individuals think of federal regulations as they affect the laboratory, they think first of the Occupational Safety and Health Administration (OSHA) standards. Although OSHA has had a significant impact on the laboratory with several important regulatory mandates, it must be understood that when establishing an effective health and safety program for a laboratory, it is not only OSHA that must be considered but also a number of other federal agencies that substantially affect the laboratory. Figure 1.1 lists the federal laws that have an impact on the medical laboratory and demonstrates the interrelationships of the various federal agencies as they relate to specific regulations. These agencies frequently interact with OSHA on health and safety issues and may also promulgate their own set of requirements.[1] If this interaction is not clearly understood, requirements may be misinterpreted when programs for regulatory compliance are developed. Another consideration should be the various agencies, commissions, or professional organizations that may issue guidelines for performance that may not be required under a particular OSHA mandate. Finally, it is important to distinguish institution or facility policies from federal mandates. When considering requirements for compliance with health and safety programs, be sure that you understand what is, in fact, a regulatory mandate, what is a guideline, and what is a policy. Be very careful when someone says "It's the law!" Is it?

Figure 1.1 FEDERAL LAWS THAT HAVE AN IMPACT ON THE MEDICAL LABORATORY

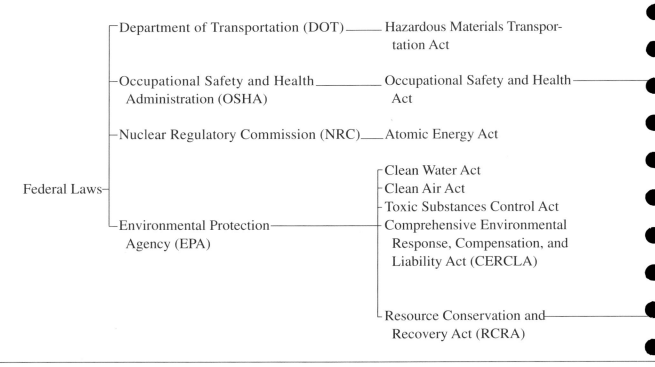

Federal Laws
- Department of Transportation (DOT) —— Hazardous Materials Transportation Act
- Occupational Safety and Health Administration (OSHA) —— Occupational Safety and Health Act
- Nuclear Regulatory Commission (NRC) —— Atomic Energy Act
- Environmental Protection Agency (EPA)
  - Clean Water Act
  - Clean Air Act
  - Toxic Substances Control Act
  - Comprehensive Environmental Response, Compensation, and Liability Act (CERCLA)
  - Resource Conservation and Recovery Act (RCRA)

(Adapted from Clinical Laboratory Waste Minimization, 1993, NCCLS Document GP-5.)

1.1.1 THE IMPACT OF OSHA STANDARDS ON LABORATORIES

A large number of individuals are employed in laboratories. The OSHA standards affect a variety of laboratory environments, primarily in the private sector (see following topics). Currently OSHA estimates this population of laboratory employees to include[2]:

- 934,000 employees in 34,214 laboratories in the United States
- 10,000 research and development laboratories
- 2500 independent industrial laboratories
- 7600 independent clinical laboratories
- 7100 hospital laboratories
- 7114 secondary and private school laboratories

1.1.2 OSHA DEFICIENCIES AND PROBLEMS

Since the original Occupational Safety and Health Act (1970), OSHA has suffered from chronic underfunding, particularly during the Reagan administration when OSHA was dealt severe cutbacks. This has caused OSHA to be less effective than other agencies such as the Environmental Protection Agency (EPA). An example of this less than equitable balance is demonstrated by the fact that OSHA receives less than $300 million to protect workers while the EPA receives $7 billion for environmental protection. (The Interior Department receives $1 billion to protect fish and wildlife alone.) OSHA has fewer than 1000 inspectors to cover 6.5

Multiple Standards Including:
- Hazard Communication Standard
- Occupational Exposure to Hazardous Chemicals in Laboratories
- The Formaldehyde Standard
- The Bloodborne Pathogen Standard
- Prevention of Transmission of Tuberculosis in the Workplace (CDC), and others

- Subtitle C: Hazardous Chemical Waste
- Subtitle D: Solid Municipal Waste
- Subtitle J: Medical (infectious and sharp) Waste

million workplaces; that is an average sighting of an inspector in the workplace every 87 years. If the facility is a high priority facility, this may be reduced to a mere 13 years.[3] (A note of caution: I would not interpret these figures to mean that compliance is not necessary because of diminished chances of being visited by an inspector. These figures are provided for illustration only.) To make matters worse, the average penalty for one serious violation is $753, while those citations levied by the EPA are estimated to be $51,329 per case (1993 figures). There are weaknesses in the OSHA laws because they have never been revised, resulting in wide disparity in protection and enforcement between the environmental and workplace laws.

1.1.3 PROPOSED OSHA REFORM

Because of serious deficiencies in OSHA, reform has been proposed,[4] which includes a number of improvements in the administration of occupational safety and health programs. Although not without opposition, the OSHA reform legislation HR1280 (1992) will probably be passed. Some important highlights of these proposals are as follows:
- Extend OSHA compliance to federal, state, and local government employees. (This is estimated to represent more than 7 million workers.)
- Initiate proactive programs to identify and correct hazards in the workplace.
- Provide a greater role for workers, including labor/management health and safety committees.
- Provide better protection from retaliation against workers.
- Substantially strengthen enforcement laws.

1.1.4 THE DIFFERENCE BETWEEN THE HAZARD COMMUNICATION AND THE OCCUPATIONAL EXPOSURES STANDARDS

The Hazard Communication and the Occupational Exposure to Hazardous Chemicals in Laboratories standards are significant because of the sizable interaction between the two mandates. Because of their focus on health and safety hazards, requirements of one apply to the other as well.[2]

1.1.4 A THE HAZARD COMMUNICATION STANDARD
This standard primarily ensures that workers know the hazards associated with chemicals in their workplace so that they can protect themselves.

1.1.4 B THE LABORATORY STANDARD
This standard requires a plan to implement practices to minimize exposures to hazardous chemicals.

1.1.5 WHAT DO THE OSHA STANDARDS HAVE IN COMMON?

OSHA health and safety–related standards have a number of requirements that are applicable or interrelated to each other. However, these standards have a number of points that are common to each, including:
- Statements of policy and implementation including dates
- Objectives of the programs
- Scope and application of the programs
- Significant terminology
- Health hazards, disease, symptoms, or signs of exposures

- Training programs and continuing education
- Standard operating procedures
- Work practices, engineering controls, and personal protective equipment (PPE)
- Exposure, incident, and follow-up procedures
- Documentation of training, medical incident, and monitoring
- Regular review, updates, and revision

1.1.6 SUGGESTED RESOURCES WHEN DEVELOPING A PROGRAM

- Create a safety resource area in your laboratory.
- Create a "form" file.
- Keep "master" copies in sleeved covers for easy access.
- Many resources are free for the asking.
- Identify what is "your" part of the program.

1.2 OSHA COVERAGE, EXCEPTIONS, AND STATE PROGRAMS[2]

In general, OSHA mandates cover all employers and employees in the 50 states, the District of Columbia, Puerto Rico, and all other territories under United States jurisdiction. Exceptions to OSHA jurisdiction include self-employed individuals, farms in which only immediate members of the employer's family are employed, workplaces protected by other federal agencies, and state and local government employees.

Many states have "private sector" plans approved by OSHA. These plans must provide a program that covers its state and local government workers and is at least as effective as its program for private employees. Presently, the states with such OSHA-approved job safety and health programs are: Alaska, Arizona, California, Connecticut (only public employees covered), Hawaii, Indiana, Iowa, Kentucky, Maryland, Michigan, Minnesota, Nevada, New Mexico, New York (only public employees covered), Oregon, Puerto Rico, South Carolina, Tennessee, Utah, Vermont, Virgin Islands, Virginia, Washington, and Wyoming.

1.2.1 THE GENERAL DUTY CLAUSE

OSHA promulgates legally enforceable standards for covered employers/employees. It is the responsibility of employers to become familiar with standards as applicable to their establishments. It is also the responsibility of employers to ensure that all employees have and use personal gear and equipment when required for safety.

Where OSHA has not promulgated a specific standard, the responsibility of the employer is to follow the Occupational Safety and Health Act of 1970 General Duty Clause, which states that each employer
- Shall furnish a place of employment which is free from recognized hazards that are causing or are likely to cause death or serious physical harm to their employees.
Therefore, lack of a specific OSHA standard does not release the employer from the legal responsibilities of protecting employees from recognized hazards.

1.3 RECORDING OCCUPATIONAL ILLNESS AND INJURY[2]

All occupational illnesses must be recorded regardless of the severity of the illness. All occupational injuries must be recorded if they result in death, one or more lost workdays, restriction of work or motion, loss of consciousness, transfer to another job, and medical treatment other than first aid. (An occupational injury is any injury such as a cut, fracture, sprain, or amputation that results from a work-related accident or from exposure involving a single incident in the workplace.)

NOTE: If an on-the-job accident occurs, which results in the death of an employee or in the hospitalization of five or more employees, all employers, regardless of the number of employees, are required to report the accident, in detail, to the nearest OSHA office within 48 hours. (Usually, the act calls for employers with 11 or more employees to maintain records of occupational illness or injury.)

1.3.1 RECORDKEEPING FORMS

Records are maintained on a year-to-year basis and must be retained for 5 years.

1.3.1 A OSHA FORM NO. 200: LOG AND SUMMARY OF OCCUPATIONAL INJURIES AND ILLNESSES
• Substitute form is acceptable with appropriate date and is easily readable.
• Injury and illness must be recorded within 6 working days of the event.

1.3.1 B OSHA FORM NO. 101: SUPPLEMENTARY RECORD OF OCCUPATIONAL INJURIES AND ILLNESSES
• Substitute forms are acceptable, as above (ie, workman's compensation forms).
• Incidents must be recorded within 6 working days of events.

1.3.2 POSTING REQUIREMENTS

A copy of the totals and information (of injuries and illness reports) for the previous year are to be posted in each facility. It must be posted no later than February 1, kept posted until March 1, and be displayed in the usual location of employee notices. Even if there were no injuries or illness to report, the information must be posted.

1.3.3 INFORMING EMPLOYEES

The following requirements must be met.
• OSHA's job safety and health protection workplace poster (form 2202 or a state equivalent) informing workers of their rights and responsibilities under the act must be posted.
• Copies of the act and copies of relevant OSHA rules and regulations must be available to employees upon request.
• Summary of any petition for variances from standard mandates or recordkeeping procedures must be kept.
• Copies of all OSHA citations for violations of standards must remain posted at or near the location of the alleged violation for 3 days, or until the violations have abated, whichever is longer.
• Log and summary of occupational injuries and illnesses (form 200) must be kept.

All employees have the right to examine any records kept by their employers regarding exposure to hazardous materials or the result of medical surveillance.

An OSHA Notice of Proposed Rulemaking (NPRM) was scheduled for late 1994 regarding the recording and reporting of occupational illnesses. The objective of this action is to simplify the recording system through revision of forms, regulations, and interpretive material, thereby increasing the reliability and utility of the information collected.

Table 1.1   RECORD RETENTION GUIDELINES*[5]

RECORD	CLIA 1988	CAP
Requisition, test	2 years	
Record, test	2 years	2 years
Report, test (preliminary & final)	2 years	2 years
Pathology test report	10 years	2 years
Quality control records	2 years	20 years
Proficiency test results	2 years	
Remedial action records (proficiency training failure)	2 years	
Instrument maintenance		Life of instrument
Test procedures	2 years	
Personnel records		
		30 years
ANATOMIC PATHOLOGY		
Histology stained slides	10 years	20 years from date of exam
Histology specimen blocks	2 years	5 years from date of exam
Histology wet tissue		2 weeks after final report
Reports	10 years	20 years
Accession log records		1 year
Maintenance records		1 year
Cytology slides	5 years	
Slides (negatives and unsatisfactory)	5 years	5 years
Slides (suspicious and positive)	5 years	20 years
Records		20 years
Accession log records		1 year
Maintenance records		2 years
Autopsy wet tissue		6 months after final report
Autopsy paraffin blocks		5 years after final report
Autopsy slides		20 years after final report
Autopsy reports		20 years after final report
Accession log records, autopsy	1 year after final report	
Maintenance records		2 years after final report

* *CLIA=Clinical Laboratories Improvement Act; CAP=College of American Pathologists.*

1.3.4 RECORD RETENTION GUIDELINES[5]

Table 1.1 is a listing of record retention guidelines.

1.3.4 A DOCUMENTS TO KEEP IN PERSONNEL FILES
- Position description
- Performance standards
- Scheduled evaluations
- Employment application
- Educational levels
- Continuing education and in-service training
- Resumé, statement of prior experience
- Training in health and safety practices
- Vaccination against hepatitis B or declination of vaccine

1.3.4 B OSHA STANDARD COMPLIANCE
Bloodborne Pathogen (1910.1030):
- Training records: 3 years from date of training
- Medical and exposure records: Employment + 30 years

Occupational Exposure to Hazardous Chemicals in Laboratories (1910.1450):
- Medical records: At least 30 years
- Environmental exposure monitoring: At least 30 years

Formaldehyde Standard (1910.1048):
- Exposure records: At least 30 years
- Medical records: Employment + 30 years
- Respirator fit test results: Until updated or changed

Benzene (1910.1028) and Specified Carcinogens (1910.1001-1016):
- Exposure monitoring: At least 30 years
- PPE: At least 30 years
- Medical surveillance: At least 30 years
- Specified carcinogens: At least 30 years

Occupational Injuries and Illness (1910.1904):
- All logs and evaluations: 5 years after end of relevant calendar year

Hazardous Waste Operations and Emergency Response:
- Medical surveillance: Employment + 30 years depending on exposure

1.3.4 C ADDITIONAL INFORMATION AND OTHER OSHA STANDARD REQUIREMENTS
Consult OSHA's generic records standard (1910.20), *Access to Medical and Exposure Records.*

1.4 BASIC GUIDELINES FOR THE OSHA INSPECTION PROCESS[2,6]

The compliance safety and health officer (CSHO) (not "inspector") conducts the inspection. There is usually a reason for the inspection. No one "just decides" to inspect a facility.

1.4.1 PROGRAMMED INSPECTIONS (SCHEDULED INSPECTIONS)

Who is selected?
- High-hazard industries
- Places with significant number of previous citations
- 5% low-hazard inspections (physicians offices and clinics)
- Facilities with 11 or more personnel
- Some random selections

1.4.2 UNPROGRAMMED INSPECTIONS

The numbers of such inspections has dramatically increased. They usually occur in response to a:
- Formal complaint, such as a signed letter or form
- Informal complaint, such as a call from an employee

Both types of complaints are kept confidential. All inspections are carried out without notice. Notice or a tip-off is illegal.

1.4.3 INSPECTION PROTOCOLS

Stringent guidelines are enforced.
Knowledgeable CSHO is assigned.
Opening conference is held with the laboratory manager, in which the manager:
- May request chemical hygiene plan.
- May request infection control plan.

Movement about the facility:
- Is conducted accompanied by employer and employee representative.
- May be accompanied by taking of photographs or video.

If complaint is specific, a "wall to wall" investigation is not carried out; however, obvious violations cannot be ignored.

Closing conference includes
- Review of all identified problems
- Reason or explanation offered by employer
- Citations issued at the site

Penalty is assessed by area director based on the following strict, established protocol:
- *Other than serious*: Failure to identify and correct ($7000)
- *Serious*: Should have known ($7000)
- *Willful*: Up to $70,000 per violation
- *Egregious*: Up to $70,000 per violation

Penalty reductions include
- 25% reduction where good intentions to correct violation exist
- 15% reduction if effective safety programs are instituted
- 10% reduction if correction is made and no previous history of citations exists

1.5 MOST COMMON VIOLATIONS

For inspections occurring during the period January through December 1992, the following were the most common violations of federal OSHA standards and the Bloodborne Pathogen Standard.

1.5.1 MOST COMMON OSHA STANDARDS VIOLATIONS

- Improper recording and reporting injuries on the OSHA form 200
- Medical and first aid: Improper use of showers following hazardous exposure
- General PPEs: Supplied, used, and maintained by employer
- Written hazard communication plan not available
- Containers not labeled with proper hazard warnings
- MSDSs not available according to Hazard Communication Standard
- Moving or hazardous parts of instrumentation: Safety guards not available
- Hazard communication training records not documented
- No hazardous energy program: Lockout/tagout
- All employment areas were not kept clean, orderly, and in sanitary conditions

1.5.2 MOST COMMON BLOODBORNE PATHOGEN VIOLATIONS

- Improper storage containers used for nonsharp waste
- Schedule and method of implementation of standard not in exposure control plan
- Inappropriate decontamination of work surfaces
- Signed declination to the hepatitis B vaccine not available
- Employee's noncompliance with use of PPE
- Hepatitis B vaccine not available
- Improper warning labels and signs used on containers of regulated waste
- Written exposure control plan not available
- Job tasks when some employees were exposed not recorded
- Improper hand washing following removal of PPEs
- Improper use of face protection
- Written schedule for cleaning and decontamination area not available
- Documentation of employee training within 90 days of standard not made
- Education on the use of engineering controls, work practices, and PPEs not documented
- Name of person conducting training not documented

1.6 THE AMERICANS WITH DISABILITIES ACT

A brief synopsis of the Americans with Disabilities Act (ADA) is included in this text, because I believe it is relevant when developing a program regarding health and safety issues. The potential concerns of the disabled should be recognized, particularly when establishing procedures involving handling, usage, or in general, manipulation of certain hazardous materials. Prominent points of the law include the following:

- The ADA provides protection and prohibits discrimination in all employment practices, including job application procedures, hiring, firing, advancement, compensation, and training of qualified employees.[7]
- The law applies to recruitment, advertising, tenure, layoff, leave, fringe benefits, and all other employment-related activities.
- The law was effective July 26, 1992, for employers with more than 25 employees and July 26, 1994, for employers with 15 to 24 employees.
- A qualified disabled person "is an individual with a disability who meets the skill, experience, education, and other job-related requirements of a position held or desired and who, with or without reasonable accommodation, can perform the essential functions of a job." [7]
- The law protects those with physical or mental impairment including those with cancer in remission, recovering drug addicts, and those with disfigurement, a live-in companion with acquired immune deficiency syndrome (AIDS) or human immunodeficiency virus (HIV), blindness, deafness, alcoholism, dyslexia, mental illness, stress, and depression.[7]

1.6.1 COMPLIANCE GUIDELINES[8]

The most important aspect of the ADA is its requirement to engage in good-faith dialogue as it relates to reasonable accommodations. The focus is on the abilities of individuals and how effective they can be at the job. The work force is growing older and working longer, and disabled employees will become more common in the future. Additional information is available from the Equal Employment Opportunity Commission by calling (800) 669-3362 or (800) 800-3302. An excellent document for reference and details of the law is the Equal Employment Opportunity Commission's *Technical Assistance Manual on the Employment Provisions (Title 1) of the ADA.*

1.6.1 A   REEVALUATION OF EXISTING JOB DESCRIPTIONS

- Job descriptions must be examined to word them to list only the essential functions of the position.
- Job requirements must be restructured without need for any or reasonable accommodations such as making a facility readily accessible to and usable by a disabled person.
- Marginal job functions must be reallocated or redistributed.
- When and how essential job functions are performed must be altered.
- Provide part-time and modified work schedules.
- Modify equipment or devices, or obtain equipment for the disabled.
- Permit use of accrued paid or unpaid leave for necessary treatment.
- Provide reserved parking for those with mobility impairments.
- Permit the use of equipment or devices that employer is not required to provide.

1.6.1 B REVIEW OF APPLICATION AND SELECTION PROCESS

- The language of applications must not be discriminatory.
- Employers cannot ask disabled applicants about the severity or nature of illness.
- Employer can ask applicants to demonstrate how they would perform essential duties of their jobs.
- Disabled applicants cannot be made to undergo a physical examination before being offered a position, but may be asked to do so after being offered the position if all other employees in that job category must do so.

1.6.1 C ACCOMMODATIONS FOR THE DISABLED

- Install appropriate ramps for wheelchairs.
- Adjust heights of bench tops.
- Acquire certain equipment or modify existing ones.
- Reschedule workers or exchange some workers' duties with others.
- Address the physical needs of the workplace, such as restrooms.
- Depending on the expense of modifications, worker must be given the opportunity to pay for at least some of the cost of accommodations.

1.6.1 D PROVISIONS FOR RETENTION OF EMPLOYEE, PROMOTIONS, AND AWARDS

Each must be based on the worker's ability to perform the essential functions of the job.

1.6.1 E EDUCATION OF SUPERVISORS AND STAFF

- Provide education and training in nondiscriminatory actions.
- Understand the contributions disabled workers can make to the laboratory.

1.7 REFERENCES

1. National Commission on Clinical Laboratory Standards. *Protection of Laboratory Workers from Infectious Disease Transmitted by Blood, Body Fluids, and Tissue.* Villanova, Pa: National Commission of Clinical Laboratory Standards. NCCLS Document M29-T2, 1991; vol 11, no 14.
2. National Training Institute. *Educational and Training Materials.* Washington, DC: Occupational Safety and Health Administration, Office of Training and Education; 1991.
3. Chapman B. OSHA inspections: not 'Seek and Destroy' missions. *CAP Today.* January 1993.
4. Smith B. OSHA reform. *Occup Health Saf.* August 1992:103.
5. Baer D. Patient records, what to save, how to save it, how long to save it. *Med Lab Observer.* February 1993:22-27.
6. Seminario P. Proposed reform of OSHA Act fulfills original objective of safe workplace. *Occup Health Saf.* September 1993:104.
7. Buccino L. Laboratory compliance with the Americans with Disabilities Act. *Adv Med Lab Prof.* August 1993.
8. Snyder J. Open your doors to the disabled: it's the law. *Med Lab Observer.* August 1992.

1.7.1　ADDITIONAL READINGS

Chapman B. Getting lab safety practices to stick. *CAP Today.* December 1992.

McNett C. Rocky road for new OSHA rules: microscope on Washington. *Lab Med.* 1992;23:641.

Seaver M. Work environments of the future promise more for the disabled. *Occup Health Saf.* September 1987.

Smith B. Health, safety professionals survive an onslaught of regulations, change. *Occup Health Saf.* June 1992:22-23.

Understanding and Compliance

Remember that the original intent or objective of the Occupational Safety and Health Administration (OSHA) standards was to provide for a safe workplace environment. Knowledge of the hazards in the workplace was originally mandated by the Hazard Communication Standard or Right-to-Know Law. The Occupational Exposures to Hazardous Chemicals in Laboratories Standard, frequently referred to as the "Laboratory Standard," significantly expands this knowledge to include methods to reduce or minimize exposures. Hazards that are included in these and other OSHA standards are: chemical hazards (both short- and long-term); biological hazards such as acquired immunodeficiency syndrome (AIDS), hepatitis B, and more recently *Mycobacterium tuberculosis*; and physical hazards which include facility environments and equipment. Compliance with these standards requires considerable planning, training, and documentation.

The success of any program depends on attitude, understanding, and action. Sincerity and enthusiasm, with a generous amount of common sense, are essential for program success.
A prominent aspect to be considered in laboratory management is that of health and safety awareness and safe laboratory practices.[1] Unfortunately, the use of good safety practices is consistently underestimated as a management tool. This is regrettable because established safety programs present several significant opportunities for effective management. These programs substantially decrease the overall economic impact on the entire laboratory operation, provide for a measurable quality control device, as well as enhance technical superiority, and finally provide personnel with the best possible physical protection while establishing an active mode of personnel participation. This participation improves program effectiveness and enhances the overall laboratory morale and enthusiasm.

Health and safety programs provide an economic advantage for several reasons. Laboratories are encouraged to purchase chemicals, reagents, or dyes only in the amounts necessary for existing work loads. Minimal use of these substances requires less storage space, special storage, or cabinet expense. This reduction of chemical supplies results in less maintenance, less inventory control, and less documentation. The overall reduction of chemical use results in considerable reduction in disposal preparation and removal expenses.

Health and safety programs provide for a technically superior product and measurable quality control. Ordering only those chemicals or dyes that are needed results in the use of fresh ingredients. Improper chemical composition and reactions are more easily observed and controlled when fresh, "known" source ingredients are used. Chemicals and dyes are exposed to less cross-contamination and decomposition when small quantities are used.

Personnel are provided with the best possible protection while being encouraged to actively participate in health and safety programs. In this manner, the confidence of the personnel in management is increased. The staff is convinced of management's sincere interest in their well-being; their active participation enhances these programs, making them more effective. Both management and staff are provided with optimal protection because personnel know what chemicals and dyes are in the laboratory, their possible hazards, and their proper use and disposal. Medical emergencies and crisis situations are anticipated and well prepared for, thereby substantially decreasing the impact of any accidents.

Finally, the overall environment and protection of scarce resources is ensured by the entire concept of "less is best," that is, consume less, be exposed to less, produce less, and dispose of less.[2] As laboratories pass into the next century and beyond, the necessity of personnel and management working closely together to effectively provide a safe and healthy workplace environment, combined with high productivity and cost-effective operations, will be increasingly important.

2.2   ORGANIZING A LABORATORY HEALTH AND SAFETY PROGRAM[1]

2.2.1   THE NEED FOR A HEALTH AND SAFETY PROGRAM

Technologists work with numerous materials with known hazards, such as
- Reactive chemicals
- Radioactive materials
- Explosive chemicals
- Biohazardous materials
- Corrosive chemicals
- Peroxidizing chemicals
- Flammable materials
- Water reactive chemicals
- Toxic chemicals
- Air reactive chemicals

Recognize that some substances considered safe today may, in the future, be found to cause unsuspected long-term disorders. Technologists are exposed to numerous physical hazards such as cuts, abrasions, and electrical shock.

2.2.2   FUNDAMENTAL ORGANIZATION OF A HEALTH AND SAFETY PLAN

There is a safe way to perform all laboratory work. Just as the concept of defensive driving can prevent accidents, adequate planning and understanding can prevent injury or illness in the laboratory.[3] The practice of safety in the laboratory requires two important factors:
- The desire of an individual for self-protection as well as concern for the protection of his or her associates
- The need to follow a set of rules

Safety morale is important because
- It is an essential part of accident and illness prevention.
- Getting everyone involved increases the effectiveness of any program.

Guidelines or rules must be established.
- There should be only a limited number of rules.
- These rules must be rigidly and impartially enforced.
- Willful noncompliance should result in a dismissal or suspension.

The supervisor should set an example by observing all the rules and being enthusiastic and sincere about health and safety issues.

Safe practice is an attitude and a knowledge of potential hazards. Many accidents are the result of an indifferent attitude and a failure to use common sense and follow instructions.

2.2.3   GENERAL SAFETY PRACTICES

2.2.3 A   ESSENTIAL SAFETY EQUIPMENT
- Safety showers
- Eye-wash stations
- Fume hoods
- Wash sinks
- Alarm systems
- Appropriate signs
- Appropriate personal protective equipment (PPE)
- Emergency telephone numbers
- Unrestricted phone
- Dry chemical powder and/or carbon dioxide fire extinguishers

2.2.3 B   FIRST AID
- Supplies and equipment must be readily available.
- Location and phone number of medical facility or physician must be accessible.

2.2.3 C   PERSONAL PROTECTIVE EQUIPMENT
- Laboratory coats and aprons
- Gloves (latex, utility, and mesh)
- Goggles, face shields, and masks
- Foot and head coverings
- Respirators where appropriate

2.2.3 D   STORAGE
Storage cabinets and appropriate carts for transport of chemicals must be safe.

2.2.3 E   DISPOSAL
- Procedures must be carefully planned to fit individual needs.
- It is an integral part of written procedures and must be carefully observed.
- Follow current regulatory guidelines and accepted practices.

2.2.3 F   INSPECTIONS
Electrical safety and routinely scheduled instrument inspections must be conducted.

2.2.4   DEFINE SPECIFIC LABORATORY SAFETY TARGETS

2.2.4 A   SAFETY TRAINING
This includes the following:
- Chemical hygiene
- Formaldehyde Standard
- Hazard Communication Standard

- Bloodborne Pathogen Standard
- Fire drills
- Use of fire extinguishers
- Chemical spills
- Biohazard spills
- Use of safety showers
- Use of eye-wash stations

2.2.4 B   EMERGENCY SITUATIONS
- What to do?
- Whom to call?
- What to do while waiting for help?

2.2.4 C   HANDLING CHEMICALS
- Reading labels
- Hazard warning systems
- Hazardous substances/chemicals
- Incompatible chemicals
- Storage
- Reactive chemicals

2.2.4 D   EQUIPMENT SAFETY
- Installation and routinely scheduled inspections
- Operation and routinely scheduled inspections
- Inspection of tubing, hoses, electrical plugs and grounds, and wiring
- Glassware such as stills
- Vacuums such as desiccators
- Fume hoods with routinely scheduled inspections

2.2.4 E   CHEMICAL SPILLS
- General safety procedures such as acid spill procedures; flammables and solvents; and caustic spill procedures
- Body contact: Large body area and confined area procedures

2.2.4 F   HAZARDOUS CHEMICALS
These include chemicals with the properties listed in 2.2.1.

2.2.4 G   HEALTH MAINTENANCE SURVEY PROGRAMS
- Recommend annual technologist evaluation
- Perform complete blood count, urinalysis, liver profile, and respiratory evaluation

2.2.5   ACTIVE ORGANIZATIONAL PLANNING

Present the health and safety program to the appropriate administrative authority.
- Discuss applicable regulatory agency mandates for compliance
- Discuss essential physical and technical requirements such as equipment and instrument needs
- Define necessary drills or demonstrations

- Discuss lecture or in-service requirements
- Suggest possible committee/personnel activity

Evaluate all recommendations and restrictions that may be given.

Present cost analysis of proposed program.

Obtain approval to proceed with the plan.

Call a general meeting to present the program and gather suggestions for implementation.
- Discuss ideas for preparation of procedure manual
- Evaluate laboratory labeling systems
- Discuss health and safety poster and signs
- Promote a health and safety-oriented bulletin board

Introduce lecture or in-service requirements and drills.
- Suggest possible guest speakers
- Encourage rotating individual or laboratory area participation in presentations
- Establish workshops, hands-on safety demonstrations and drills
- Organize and designate necessary committees, committee members, and/or laboratory representatives

2.2.6   GATHER RESOURCES AND INFORMATION

Recognize not only when to get help but where to find answers to your problems. Awareness and safety planning emphasize the need for adequate safety precautions, such as the need for training in laboratory environments and increased awareness of health effects of exposures.

Safety awareness is a subject of such magnitude that it can be beyond the scope and resources of most institutions. Individuals are urged to seek specific guidance from appropriate federal and state agencies and specialized textbooks concerning health and safety.

Resource material for health and safety programs includes:
- National Institute for Occupational Safety and Health guidelines for health and safety
- OSHA federal standards and guidelines
- Professional journals
- National Fire Protection Agency publications
- Professional organizations and newsletters
- Area Poison Control Boards
- Regional OSHA offices
- Local fire department and related safety agencies/offices
- Colleges and university resources
- Medical schools or regional medical centers
- Communication with colleagues

2.2.7 ESTABLISH A HEALTH AND SAFETY RESOURCE AREA

- Include copies of all appropriate OSHA standards
- Include facility chemical hygiene plan
- Include facility infection control plan
- Establish and maintain current file of publications/articles relating to health and safety issues
- Provide current material safety data sheet, manufacturers' instructions, warnings, or updates
- Provide current reference books, charts, and information data
- Provide a current and constantly updated health and safety procedure manual that includes the appropriate information such as fire drills and safety inspections

2.2.8 IDENTIFY HEALTH AND SAFETY ISSUES IN THE LABORATORY

- Identify OSHA standards and other regulatory agency mandates that apply to the laboratory
- Identify guidelines that may affect the laboratory such as the National Fire Protection Agency and American National Standards Institute guidelines
- Identify the use of PPE in the laboratory
- Describe the hazards associated with compressed gases and flammable liquids
- Evaluate the ventilation systems of the laboratory
- Describe the emergency response program for the laboratory
- Describe the procedures for actual hazards, accidents, exposures, or injury
- Describe the evaluation and follow-up of accidents, exposures, and injury
- Identify hazards in the laboratory that are associated with the use of chemicals, biological hazards, and physical or ergonomic concerns

2.2.9 ASSESSMENT OF HEALTH AND SAFETY PROGRAMS

- Does the program address the full range of hazards found in the workplace?
- Is the program written in a clearly defined and easily understood manner?
- Are all workers provided education and training regarding the program?
- Do all workers have access to the written program?
- Are workers informed by use of posters, signage, labels, or other means?
- Are routinely scheduled health and safety meetings for all workers part of the program?
- Is there a trainer or knowledgeable leader guiding these meetings?
- Are the program mandates reviewed regularly for compliance?
- Are the program mandates enforced and, if so, by what methods?
- Are accidents, exposures, injuries, or illnesses investigated and preventive measures determined?
- Are specific health hazards identified and methods of monitoring hazards described?
- Is there a comprehensive medical surveillance program established, which covers all employees and describes methods of testing, when testing is performed, and by whom?
- Are engineering and administrative controls described in detail?
- Is PPE provided with requirements for selection, use, and maintenance?

2.3 THE BLIND FISH FACTOR

An incident occurs in the laboratory that "should just not have happened"; all guidelines, work practices, and engineering controls were in place, and personnel had been adequately and thoroughly trained. Situations such as this leave administrators wondering not only why it occurred but also how to prevent future occurrences. The cause of an accident is not carelessness, distraction, or laziness but the "blind fish factor." Cave-dwelling fish adapt to the dark and cannot see to protect themselves from predators when suddenly swimming into a lighted pool; similarly, laboratory workers become accustomed to routine situations in the laboratory and sometimes cannot prevent accidents from happening.[4]

2.3.1 THE BLIND FISH FACTOR IN THE LABORATORY

In the laboratory, a sense of false security becomes established: "It has not happened to me before, therefore nothing will occur now." This may be true as long as the environment remains the same, but the unexpected event can turn a situation into disaster ("I've mixed these chemicals together a million times before with no problem"). When tasks are performed routinely, the laboratory worker begins to eliminate certain aspects of the procedure that are perceived as inefficient. This action has potential problems if the situation changes (eg, forgetting to wear gloves when handling a potentially infectious specimen). When attempts are made to correct this behavior, such as confronting the individual concerning the action, the individual will stop momentarily, but soon begin the process again. Rewriting procedures, developing guidelines, and issuing ultimatums are only temporary (Band-Aid) solutions.

2.3.2 MEASURES TO PREVENT THE BLIND FISH FACTOR[4]

- Adaptability is everyone's concern. Take actions to prevent the potential harmful effects.
- Set high standards of performance.
- Keep safety issues in the forefront using complements, simulations, retraining, and testing.
- Develop personal check systems to prevent problem areas of performance such as asking "Is there something I stopped doing that I should be doing."
- Double-check your activities. Use a buddy system of peer observation.
- Be sure that you are up-to-date when performing procedures that you have not done in a while and may only half remember.
- Establish and develop repetition in job habits. Constant proper repetition in a task helps to ensure correct performance.
- Redesign workstations or jobs so as to provide for minimum interruption of the habit flow. This action will improve habit retention.
- Develop scenarios to maintain habits through a disruption.
- Create nonstandard environments or situations, and practice drills in, unusual situations.
- Remember that survival means adapting to prevailing conditions.

2.4 ERGONOMICS IN THE LABORATORY

Ergonomics is the science of adapting the working environment to the anatomic, physiologic, and psychological characteristics of personnel to enhance their efficiency and well-being. Unfortunately, ergonomics is usually not considered during design or selection of work systems until something goes wrong. An increased concern in the laboratory regarding cumulative trauma disorders such as carpal tunnel syndrome, tendonitis, epicondylitis (tennis elbow), thoracic outlet compression syndrome (brachial neuritis), trigger finger, and Raynaud's syndrome (a peripheral vascular disease) has caused laboratories to address the problems of workplace system design.[5] Laboratories must consider not only the health and well-being of personnel but also the potential liability of inappropriate workstation and workplace systems. From reports accumulated in 1991, the average back injury resulted in compensations of $7400, whereas the average upper body cumulative trauma disorder resulted in compensations of over $15,400.[6]

2.4.1 METHODS OF SYSTEM DESIGN[7]

Determine objectives and performance specifications of the job tasks.
Define the system or procedure to be accomplished:
- The functions and tasks to be performed
- The interrelationship between other functions or tasks

Design/determine function allocation:
- Human capabilities and limitations

Interface design with the rest of the system or operation.
- Optimize human performance.
- Minimize error risk or injury.
- Emphasize physical dimension of workstations to encourage natural posture and movement.

Facilitate design
- What materials are needed for the operation?
- What procedure manuals, training, or performance aids are needed?
- Does the design target the user and not the process?

Test and evaluate performance
- Are there mechanisms to measure personnel, equipment, and procedure performance?
- Is equipment purchased with consideration of operator performance needs and does it interface with existing systems?

2.4.2 DETERMINING SPECIFIC CORRECTIVE MEASURES[8]

- Understand that quick fixes do not work. Wrist rests and back cushions may provide temporary relief but problems continue and usually get worse.
- Observe that similar symptoms may have different causes for different people. No two people perform the same task in the same way.

- Avoid repetitive motion stress, which can contribute to cumulative trauma disorders, whenever possible, by providing regular breaks from the routine or rotation of the job task among personnel.
- Avoid chairs that have arm rests that are too high causing "hunched" posture and exaggerated angles between arm and shoulders which can contribute to brachial neuritis compression syndrome.
- Redesign workstations or procedures to prevent wrists being so close to the body as to force arms to be close to and bump against the body, such as in keyboards.
- Avoid procedures that result in twisting, bending, lifting, or any awkward or unnatural positioning of the body.
- Avoid nonadjustable chairs.
- Provide appropriate back support.
- Provide appropriate floor mats or cushioned mats for long-term, standing requirements.
- Provide appropriate, nonglare, nonreflecting light sources.

2.4.3   OSHA GUIDELINES FOR PROCESS SAFETY[9]

OSHA *Process Safety Management of Highly Hazardous Chemicals* (29 CFR 1910.119, July 1990;55[137]) states that "the process hazard analysis shall address the human factor." A new OSHA standard, "A National Ergonomics Safety Standard," is currently being developed. The Ergonomic Protection Standard proposed rule is expected to be released in Fall 1994. Following the draft "Ergonomic Protection Standard: Summary of Key Provisions" (June 1994), the performance-oriented standard is written in straightforward, simple language and will contain certain of the following key provisions:

- *Implementation*: A phase-in period for compliance will be scheduled.
- *Scope and Application*: Musculoskeletal disorders occur in all workplaces and the application of the standard depends on the extent of worker problems. (Carpal tunnel syndrome is a well-documented illness among histotechnologists and computer vision syndrome is becoming an increasing problem among those workers who use computers extensively.)
- *Documentation*: Employers must implement a procedure for receiving and responding to employee reports of risk factors or musculoskeletal problems or injuries.
- *Education*: Employers must provide information and training concerning musculoskeletal disorders.
- *Identification* of Potential Problems: OSHA Log 200 and/or symptom surveys must be used to determine whether any musculoskeletal injuries or illnesses have occurred during the past 2 years. A sample survey form will the included in the standard.
- *Survey Checklist*: A checklist will also be included with the standard and will be used to determine whether certain risk factors warrant action. Risk factors such as repetitive work processes, duration of work processes, work posture, or other significant factors must be considered. Risk factors such as hand force, awkward postures, temperature extremes (hot or cold), poor lighting and workstation design will also have to be considered. Duration of work processes will be set in measures such as 5 to 59 minutes, 1 to 4 hours, and more than 4 hours.
- *Problem Correction*: When any problem is determined with a job process, the employer is required to correct the situation or problem.
- *Employee Involvement and Training*: Workers must be actively involved in all stages of the ergonomic process. Training is required for all workers involved in potential risk jobs.

- *Medical Evaluation*: Workers with musculoskeletal problems must be evaluated by an appropriate health care provider. Appropriate treatment and follow-up must be provided. The standard will contain an appendix to assist health care professionals in their evaluations and documentation.
- *Program Evaluation*: Employers must implement a plan to determine effectiveness of their program and their ability to correct problems. The standard will provide information that employers can use to determine if they are in compliance with the standard.

2.5 COMPUTER VISION SYNDROME

An estimated 10 million workers in the United States suffer from some form of computer vision syndrome. The increasing concern for individuals who are engaged in intense computer use for more than 2 hours a day has prompted a number of studies to address the problem. Symptoms displayed by video display terminal (VDT) users include multiple vision problems such as eye strain; blurred vision; temporary myopia (nearsightedness); dry, irritated eyes; neck and backache; photophobia (sensitivity to light); double vision; and afterimages. Considering the increasing number of computer applications in laboratories, it is important to provide appropriate guidelines for computer use.

2.5.1 PRACTICES CONTRIBUTING TO COMPUTER VISION SYNDROME

- Improper lighting, reflection, and glare
- Unique or improper viewing angles
- Inappropriate distance from VDT or hard copy
- Improper spectacle design especially for farsighted individuals over age 40 years
- High VDT placement
- Poor VDT resolution
- Poor workstation design and setting

2.5.2 MEASURES TO PREVENT COMPUTER VISION SYNDROME[10]

- Take 5- to 10-minute "vision breaks" every 2 hours of continuous VDT use. Relax eyes by focusing on objects at least 20 feet away.
- Place document holder so that hard copy is at the same height and place as the VDT.
- Sit at least 16 to 30 inches away from the VDT.
- Place the VDT about 5 to 6 inches below eye level.
- Facility windows should be at right angles to the VDT, never in front.
- Provide enough light for easily reading hard copy while reducing overall lighting. Eliminate overhead or desk light reflection.
- Make sure VDT has a sharp picture contrast.
- Use antiglare filter for VDT screen. VDT-related products that have passed specifications for reduced glare are now approved by the American Optometric Association seal.

2.6 REFERENCES

1. Montgomery L. *Understanding the Right-to-Know Law, Education and Training Manual.* Baton Rouge, La: Louisiana State University School of Veterinary Medicine; 1988.
2. Task Force on RCRA. *Less is Better, Laboratory Chemical Management for Waste Reduction.* Washington, DC: Department of Government Relations, American Chemical Society; 1985.
3. American Chemical Society. *Safety in the Academic Chemistry Laboratories.* 3rd ed. Washington, DC: American Chemical Society; 1984.
4. Hazel K. Work habits can evolve dangerously according to blind fish factor. *Occup Health Saf.* October 1993:79-82.
5. Gervais P. Ergonomics part I: cumulative trauma disorder and carpal tunnel syndrome. *The Network.* November 1993;XI(4).
6. Fieger S. Human factor analysis useful for process safety management. *Occup Health Saf.* March 1993:25-32.
7. Mahone D. Review of system designs employs ergonomics prior to work injuries. *Occup Health Saf.* May 1993:89-105.
8. Chong I. Prioritize office workstation goals and watch out for 'voodoo ergonomics'. *Occup Health Saf.* October 1993:55-59.
9. Smith B. OSHA releases ergonomics draft. *Occup Health Saf.* September 1994:10.
10. Von Stroh R. Computer vision syndrome. *Occup Health Saf.* October 1993:62-66.

Chapter 3

The Hazard Communication Standard

The "Right-to-Know" Law

3.1 EDUCATION AND TRAINING PROGRAM[1]

There are approximately 25 million employees who are exposed to one or more chemicals in the workplace. There are an estimated 575,000 existing chemicals or chemical products and hundreds of new ones that are being introduced each year. These statistics, according to the Occupational Safety and Health Administration (OSHA), pose a serious health hazard for exposed individuals. Therefore, the hazard communication or Right-to-Know Law was promulgated.[2]

3.1.1 TRAINING[3]

Training programs for the Right-to-Know Law contain information regarding chemicals or other hazards in the workplace including:
- The chemical and common names of the substance
- The location of the substance in the workplace
- Proper and safe handling practices
- First-aid treatment and antidotes in case of exposure
- Adverse health effects or hazards of the substance
- Procedures for leak or spill clean-up
- Characteristics of the substance, such as flammability, explosiveness, and reactivity
- The rights of employees under the Right-to-Know Law

3.1.2 EMPLOYEE RIGHTS

All employees have the following rights under the Right-to-Know Law (Figure 3.1):
- The right to know of the listed hazardous substances present in the workplace
- The right to obtain copies of a material safety data sheet (MSDS) for each hazardous substance present
- The right to refuse to work, under certain circumstances, with a hazardous substance, if a copy of the MSDS is not provided within 3 working days after a written request for information is made (Figure 3.2)
- The right to instruction, within 30 days of employment, and at least annually thereafter, on the adverse effects of each hazardous substance with which they work, how to use each substance safely, and what to do in an emergency (Figure 3.3)
- The right to obtain additional information on the properties and effects of a hazardous substance
- The right of protection against retaliation, discharge, discipline, or discrimination as the result of exercising any of these rights

3.1.3 EMPLOYEE RESPONSIBILITIES

Any institution operates more effectively with informed people. Therefore, it is only appropriate that institutions want all employees to be informed. Employees are expected to assist in maintaining safe workplace environments by observing the precautions stated in the MSDS and utilizing the information and protective measures as instructed.

Figure 3.1 THE RIGHT-TO-KNOW LAW

You have the
RIGHT-TO-KNOW
about hazardous substances in the workplace!

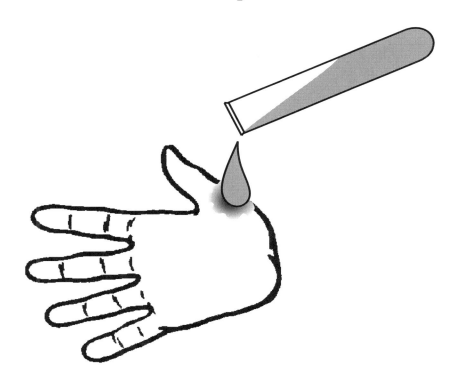

Contact your Supervisor for more information. The Right-to-Know Law* is for your safety and protection!

*The OSHA Hazard Communication Standard

3.1.4 EMPLOYER RESPONSIBILITIES

The employer has the responsibility to notify all employees that they may request information and to provide that information within 3 working days upon written request. The employer must educate and train employees in safe and proper handling of hazardous substances in the workplace. The employer must maintain records of employee exposures and records of training.

Figure 3.2 EMPLOYEE INFORMATION REQUEST FORM

Name _____ Job Title _____

Work Location/Section _____ Area/Room No. _____

Supervisor _____ Phone _____

DESCRIBE briefly the substance that you are exposed to or request information about:

Trade Name _____

Chemical Name/ Ingredients _____

Chemical Formula _____ Manufacturer/Source _____

Order/Catalog No. _____ Phone _____

Attach a label or copy of complete label information. If there is no label, state so, and describe the situation:
_____

Is there any other information which will identify the substance?
_____

If there has been an exposure to this substance, describe the circumstances of this exposure:
_____

Do you have specific questions regarding this substance?
_____

Requested by _____ Date _____

Received by _____ Date _____ Time _____

Copy of Information Attached [ ]   Request Completed [ ]

Employee Signature _____ Date _____ Time _____

Supervisor _____ Date _____

3.2 MATERIAL SAFETY DATA SHEETS

Most of the information needed for protection against chemical substance hazards is to be found in the MSDS for that substance. Each department or facility (depending on size of the institution) has the MSDS on file for each chemical used in the workplace. As responsible employees, everyone is expected to review this material.

The MSDS is a formal document that contains information about the properties and hazards of a chemical or substance. It has become an important part of health and safety programs. The original MSDS was mandated by the Hazard Communication Standard (1985) and the Occupational Exposures to Chemicals in Laboratories Standard (1990). The Environmental Protection Agency (EPA) also requires the MSDS for all emergency and response officials under their guidelines.

Because of many complaints regarding the original MSDS format, action has been taken to standardize this valuable information. Many users have commented that no two sheets looked alike. Even on the same chemical, sheets from different manufacturers may have a completely different appearance, format, symbols, size, and overall style. The sheets were frequently difficult to read, particularly in emergency situations and, in general, tended to be very confusing.

Figure 3.3 RECORD OF TRAINING

This is to certify that I have read the Employee Right-to-Know Information and have had instruction and training concerning hazardous substances in the workplace. I have had instruction and training concerning those hazards that pertain to my job, work area, and department.

| Employee Signature | SS No. | Department | Date |

This is to certify that I have discussed the right to know and policies that pertain to their job, work area, and department with this employee.

| Supervisor/Department Head Signature | | Date |

Additional Training

| Employee | Initials | Supervisor | Date |

The American National Standards Institute (ANSI) approved the new standard for MSDS in June 1993.[4] The standard represents the basic information needed for manufacturers of chemicals to develop and format a consistent MSDS that is easy to read and comprehend. Working together, the Chemical Manufacturers Association (CMA) and the ANSI have reached a consensus on this new format, which recognizes four significant factors regarding chemical usage.

- What is the material and what do users need to know about the material?
- What should a user do if a hazardous situation occurs?
- How can a user prevent a hazardous situation from occurring?
- Is there other useful information that users should know about the material?

Table 3.1 lists the major differences between the old and new MSDS forms. The ANSI has expanded the format to include information that may not apply within the United States but is required internationally. Information that is internationally applied may not necessarily be included in the MSDS per se but rather as supplements to the MSDS provided, whereby data are supplied to users through information bulletins or a list of telephone numbers. Because one of the primary uses of the MSDS is for emergency responders, this information has been included first on the new form. Other recommendations for the new form include avoiding the

Table 3.1 COMPARISON OF THE NEW AND OLD MATERIAL SAFETY AND DATA SHEET (MSDS) FORMS

NEW MSDS FORM	OLD MSDS FORM
1. Identification	1. Chemical identity
2. Composition and ingredients information	2. Hazardous ingredients
3. Hazards identification	3. Physical and chemical characteristics
4. First-aid procedures	4. Fire and explosion hazards
5. Fire fighting procedures	5. Health hazards
6. Accidental release measures	6. Reactivity
7. Exposure control (personal protective equipment)	7. Protective equipment and handling
8. Handling and storage	8. Control measures, spill, and leak
9. Physical and chemical properties	9. Handling and storage
10. Stability and reactivity information	10. Special information

INTERNATIONAL INFORMATION

11. Toxicological information
12. Ecological information
13. Disposal guidelines
14. Transport information
15. Regulatory information and consideration
16. Other information

use of Roman numerals; specific margin formats; spacing between sections; using recognized printing styles; avoiding the use of color highlighting; avoiding symbols and signs wherever possible; and very significantly, using simple sentences in the active person, eliminating footnotes and margin notes, and avoiding the use of technical language and jargon.

The standard contains samples of the MSDS, commonly used phrases, and their appropriate sections, references, and a glossary. (Another standard on computer applications [ANSI ACS X12.36] is also available.) Information on these standards can be obtained by contacting the ANSI, 655 15th Street NW, Suite 300, Washington, DC 20005, or the CMA, 2501 M Street NW, Washington, DC 20005.

Users who have accumulated notebooks of MSDS in compliance with the existing standard are still required to maintain the original MSDS information because it is applicable to personnel already working under ANSI-issued guidelines. Collection of the new MSDSs will be a gradual and on-going process.[5] The ANSI is not a regulatory agency and this new proposed form is, therefore, not a regulatory mandate. Manufacturers are not mandated to place this form into production. Considering the enormous effort and expense of generating the original MSDS mandate, manufacturers may be slow to implement this new format into their product information (Richard Dapson, personal communication).[5]

3.2.1 LETTER REQUESTING AN MSDS

Obtaining MSDSs on all hazardous chemicals used in the laboratory is a significant requirement of the hazard communication standard. From time to time, it may be necessary to request information from the manufacturer of a particular substance. Figure 3.4 is an example of a straightforward request letter that can be used to obtain the necessary MSDS to complete your records.

3.3 CHEMICAL INFORMATION[6]

3.3.1 WHAT YOU NEED TO KNOW ABOUT A CHEMICAL

Whether you are referring to the original MSDS form or the new proposed ANSI format, there is certain information that the laboratory should have readily available with regard to any chemical use.

3.3.1 A CHEMICAL (PRODUCT) NAME AND IDENTIFICATION

Chemical Abstract Service Registry number which identifies the chemical; EPA number assigned to the chemical; generic name, trade name, or synonyms; the chemical formula and other identity information; and hazard severity/predominant hazard.

3.3.1 B HAZARDOUS INGREDIENTS OF THE CHEMICAL OR MIXTURE

Material and percent of the mixture; nature of the hazard; and toxicity data including significant animal studies.

3.3.1 C PHYSICAL DATA

Boiling point; vapor pressure; vapor density; solubility in water; melting point; specific gravity; percentage of volatile volume; evaporation rate; appearance; and odor threshold.

3.3.1 D FIRE AND EXPLOSION HAZARDS

Flash point; lower explosion level (LEL); upper explosion level (UEL); flammable (signal words); and special equipment or fire fighting procedures.

3.3.1 E HEALTH HAZARDS

Threshold limit value (TLV); permissible exposure limit (PEL); routes of exposure; and how the chemical may enter the body.

Figure 3.4 EXAMPLE OF A LETTER REQUESTING AN MSDS

Date _____

RE: Request for MSDS on your product _____ Catalog No. _____

Because the Occupational Safety and Health Administration (OSHA) Hazard Communication Standard (29 CFR 1910.1200) as well as other applicable federal laws and regulations requires us to obtain material safety data sheets (MSDSs) for all hazardous substances used in our laboratory, we are requesting a copy of the MSDS for this product. We are also requesting any additional information, supplemental MSDSs, or any other relevant data that your company or supplier has concerning the safety and health aspects of this product.

Please consider this letter as a standing request to your company to forward any update information concerning the safety and health aspects of using this product.

Send the requested information to:

(Address)

Thank you for your consideration and immediate response to this request. If you have any questions concerning this matter, please do not hesitate to contact me.

Sincerely,

3.3.1 F REACTIVITY

Description of reactivity potential of the chemical; conditions to avoid during handling, use, storage, and disposal; toxic substances emitted from reaction; stability; and decomposition and the conditions under which it may occur.

3.3.1 G PERSONAL PROTECTIVE EQUIPMENT

Equipment that is necessary and ventilation requirements for use.

3.3.1 H SPILL AND LEAK PROTECTION

Specific steps to be taken; disposal methods of excess or spilled material; and other precautions or protective equipment.

3.3.1 I HANDLING AND STORAGE

A detailed written narrative should be provided.

3.3.1 J SPECIAL INFORMATION

Any precaution or directions not given previously such as any recommendations for medical surveillance and annual examinations.

3.3.2 CHEMICAL PRODUCTS OR SUBSTANCES

Because of the vast numbers of chemicals, it would be impossible to list each chemical and its related hazard in a general training program. Each section or work unit should contact its safety officer concerning specific chemicals in that area.

3.3.3 ORGANIC SOLVENTS

Organic chemicals and solvents are very commonly used in laboratories. Most organic solvents affect the central nervous system and the skin. The principal modes of exposure are inhalation of vapor and skin contact. Excessive solvent vapor inhalation may cause impairments that have no immediate discernible permanent effects on health. Immediate effects of excessive inhalation, such as lack of coordination or drowsiness, however, may increase the risk of accidents.

Other solvent exposures (eg, benzene) may result in serious impairments such as cancer or damage to the bone marrow, blood, lungs, liver, kidney, and gastrointestinal tract.

Miscellaneous solvents include nitroparaffins, certain vegetable origin solvents, and carbon disulfide, one of the most dangerous solvents used. These may cause permanent damage to the central and peripheral nervous systems and are highly flammable. Even the most inert solvents can dissolve the skin's natural protective barriers of fats and oils and leave the skin unprotected and vulnerable to dermatitis and infection. Skin contact with solvents may cause dermatitis, which may range from minor irritation to severe damage to the skin. Oils and similar substances clog the skin's pores and can cause severe eruptions if good personal hygiene practices are not followed. Certain oils, similar to hydraulic fluids, may contain substances that are highly toxic if ingested or inhaled.

Personal hygiene practices include washing all exposed areas thoroughly, drying the area completely, and changing laboratory coats or clothes as appropriate.

3.3.4 CLASSIFICATIONS OF SOLVENTS

3.3.4 A   HYDROCARBONS
- All solvents in this group are flammable.
- Most have a narcotic effect, and excessive exposure can lead to loss of muscular coordination, collapse, and unconsciousness.
- Chronic exposure to benzene may result in leukemia.

3.3.4 B   HALOGENATED HYDROCARBONS
- This group of solvents is dangerous to liver and kidneys (eg, carbon tetrachloride).
- Chlorinated naphthalenes damage the liver, causing toxic jaundice.
- Many solvents in this group have NO known toxic effect.

3.3.4 C   ALCOHOLS
- Produce mildly toxic effects on inhalation.
- Methyl alcohol may cause blindness if ingested. It is a poison.
- May constitute a serious fire hazard because of their low flash point.

3.3.4 D   ETHERS
- Highly flammable, can be explosive
- Strong narcotic properties
- Mildly toxic for the most part

3.3.4 E   GLYCOL DERIVATIVES
- Flammable
- Narcotic, and have a toxic effect on the nervous system and blood

3.3.4 F   KETONES
- Highly flammable
- Very irritating effects on nose, eyes, and upper respiratory tract. Do not inhale vapors if possible.

3.3.5 OXIDIZING SUBSTANCES

Oxidizing substances may be classified, depending on their use, as neutral, alkaline, or acidic compounds. In liquid and vapor form, these substances not only cause skin burns but are very irritating to eyes, mucous membranes, and respiratory tract. Highly toxic substances, such as hydrofluoric acid, are strongly corrosive, highly irritating, and poisonous. Nose bleeds and sinus problems have been associated with exposure to low levels of fluoride or chlorine in the air. Oxidizing substances are highly dangerous because of their ability to ignite combustible materials. The peroxides of potassium and sodium react vigorously with water and release oxygen and high levels of heat. If combustible materials are present, fire is likely to occur.

Chlorates and inorganic nitrates are strongly oxidizing substances and can cause not only fire but also explosion when mixed with finely divided combustible material such as certain dusty forms of floor sweepings. Table 3.2 lists some frequently used oxidizing substances.

3.3.6 PYROTECHNIC CHEMICALS

Fire and explosion are immediate dangers. These include: (1) combustible materials such as resins, gums, shellac, sulfur, and flake aluminum; (2) oxidizing materials such as potassium chlorate and barium chlorate; (3) flame tinting materials such as barium carbonate, sodium oxalate, Paris green; and (4) inert material such as paraffin and lime.

3.3.6 A HANDLING

Finely divided metals, like flake aluminum, should be stored in closed containers. Moisture and dampness enhance spontaneous combustions and if the metals become wet, fire, and explosion may occur. Quantities of these substances should be limited when mixing or processing.

3.3.6 B HEALTH HAZARDS

These include skin contact and inhalation of dusts and toxic materials, usually lead compounds. Respirators should be worn during mixing.

3.3.7 CORROSIVE MATERIALS

Substances listed in Table 3.3 are very serious health hazards and should be handled with great care.

3.3.7 A HEALTH HAZARDS OF CORROSIVES
- Acids and alkalis may produce respiratory irritation.
- Inhalation of many gaseous or volatile compounds produce narcotic effects.
- Metabolic disturbances occur due to the absorption of certain complex organic compounds.

Table 3.2 FREQUENTLY USED OXIDIZING SUBSTANCES

Copper chloride	Sulfuric acid
Sodium sulfide	Hydrogen peroxide
Stannous dichloride	Potassium chloride
Iodine in potassium iodide	Potassium iodate
Iodine in potassium hydroxide	Perchloric acid

Table 3.3 CORROSIVE CHEMICALS IN THE LABORATORY

Hydrazine	Sodium hypochlorate
Ammonia	Hydrochloric acid
Sodium hydroxide	Tribasic sodium phosphates
Caustic alkalies	Sodium hexametaphosphate
Calcium hydroxide	Phosphate and sulfonate based detergents
Chromic acid	

- Skin dermatitis condition known as "chrome holes" can occur; ulcers most commonly found on the hands and nose, can be caused by chromic acid.

3.4 HAZARDOUS WASTE MANAGEMENT PROGRAM

3.4.1 PURPOSE

A hazardous waste management program is responsible for adopting, implementing, and monitoring all hazardous substances that may be used in the laboratory or institution depending on the size and circumstances of the facility. Responsible individuals will meet on a regular basis and will be charged with all regular and periodic activities concerning the handling and disposal of all hazardous substances. The hazardous waste management program will keep abreast of all new laws and regulatory developments that occur regarding hazardous substances in the workplace.

3.4.2 FUNCTION

- Develop written policies and procedures concerning hazardous waste.
- Establish safe rules and practices in all departments concerning hazardous waste.
- Make available to all employees upon request information that explains the properties and hazards of each hazardous substance that they may have been exposed to.

3.4.3 DEFINITIONS

3.4.3 A WASTE
A product or material that is no longer needed and is discarded in some fashion. If you keep a material for further use, or recycle the material, it is not a waste.

3.4.3 B HAZARDOUS WASTE
As defined by the federal government, this is waste that is toxic, corrosive, ignitable, or reactive. Such materials may have a low flash point, are either extremely acidic or alkaline, can explode or react violently, or have specific components at specified levels.

3.4.3 C EMPLOYEE ASSISTANCE
Employees who need information on toxic or hazardous substances. Request forms for such information are to be provided.

3.4.4 ACCIDENTS OR INCIDENCE REPORTS

All accidents or incidents concerning hazardous waste should be documented by the immediate supervisor on an accident or incident report form and followed up by appropriate procedures or individuals.

3.5 SECTION-SPECIFIC OR DEPARTMENTAL EMERGENCY MEDICAL INFORMATION FILE

Depending on the size and organization of a facility, it may be helpful to establish a section-specific or departmental personnel emergency information file (Figure 3.5). If an accidental injury or sudden illness should occur, this file could save valuable time in seeking treatment for personnel, providing instant information without having to search through other records.

3.6 SUMMARY

The Hazard Communication Standard has had a dramatic impact on the laboratory environment since it became law in 1988. As readers proceed to the next chapter on the

Figure 3.5 EMERGENCY MEDICAL INFORMATION

(This information is confidential and is provided on a volunteer basis for personnel who wish to participate in the Emergency Medical Information program for our laboratory.)

Date _____

Name _____ Age _____ SS# _____

Address _____

IN CASE OF EMERGENCY CALL: _____

Relation _____ Phone _____

Doctor _____ Phone _____

Hospital Preference _____ Phone _____

Blood Type _____ Known Allergies _____ Drug Allergies _____

Known Medical Conditions _____

Are you on any medications? _____

Additional Comment: _____

I give my permission for this information to be given to ambulance personnel or other responsible individual in the event of a medical emergency.

Signed _____ Date _____

Occupational Exposures to Hazardous Chemicals in Laboratories Standard, they will recognize how these two laws overlap in some places and actually appear to be contradictory in others. Any discrepancies not clearly understood should be followed through by a call to the local OSHA regional office for clarification. For emphasis and summary, however, the Hazard Communication Standard presents a clearly defined program of hazard communication including all the steps outlined in Table 3.4.

Table 3.4 THE HAZARD COMMUNICATION STANDARD: A SUMMARY

BEGIN BY TAKING THE FOLLOWING STEPS

Post a notice telling employees that they have the right to know.

Take an inventory of hazardous substances in the laboratory.

Obtain MSDSs on all hazardous substances.

Plan a program to provide appropriate training.

Keep records of training and exposures.

EMPLOYEE RIGHTS

All requests for and must receive all requested chemical information *must be complied with.*

The employee may refuse to work if information is not received within 72 hours.

Exercise the right-to-know without fear of reprisal.

File a complaint if reprisals are forthcoming.

EMPLOYER RESPONSIBILITIES

Notify workers that they may request information; provide same upon request.

Train employee in safe and proper handling of hazardous substances.

Keep records of employee exposures.

NOTIFICATION AND INFORMATION

A sign must be posted to inform employees about the right to know.

Information must be made available in writing.

Information must be maintained and updated as appropriate.

Written information must be provided to employee upon request within 72 hours.

EDUCATION AND TRAINING

Employer provides training program for regularly exposed employees.

Staff must be educated and trained with regard to safety procedures and inherent dangers before initial assignment of job and at least annually thereafter.

3.7 REFERENCES

1. Hazard Communication Standard; Final Rule, 29 CFR Parts 1910.1915, 1917, 1918, 1926, and 1928. Washington, DC: Department of Labor, Occupational Safety and Health Administration; 1987:31852-31886.
2. Montgomery L. *Understanding the Right-to-Know Law, Education and Training Manual.* Baton Rouge, La: Louisiana State University School of Medicine; 1988.
3. OSHA National Training Institute. *Laboratory Safety and Health.* Des Plaines, Ill: Occupational Safety and Health Administration, Office of Training and Education; 1991. Course Material No. 224.
4. Luebbert P. New MSDS standard welcome. *Adv Med Lab Prof.* September 10, 1993:11.
5. Montgomery L. New MSDS forms proposed. *The Network.* 1994;11(1).
6. Snow J, ed. *Handling of Carcinogens and Hazardous Chemicals.* LaJolla, Calif: Calibochemical; 1982.

3.7.1 ADDITIONAL READINGS

American Chemical Society. *Less is Better, Laboratory Chemical Management for Waste Reduction.* Washington, DC: American Chemical Society; 1985.

American Chemical Society. *Safety in Academic Chemistry Laboratories.* 3rd ed. Washington, DC: American Chemical Society; August 1979.

Committee on Hazardous Substances in the Laboratory, National Research Council. *Prudent Practices for Disposal of Chemicals from Laboratories.* Washington, DC: National Academy Press; 1983.

Committee on Hazardous Substances in the Laboratory, National Research Council. *Prudent Practices for Disposal of Chemicals from Laboratories.* Washington, DC: National Academy Press; 1985.

Feldman A. You and the right-to-know law. *Lipshaw Lableader.* Spring 1985;2(2):1,5.

Fragula G. Handling hazardous materials in the hospital laboratory. *J Histotechnol.* March 1984;7(1):15-19.

Howard B. Laboratory safety: more important than ever. *J Histotechnol.* 1986;9(1):25-26.

Lane D. Taking charge of your inventory. *Vet Econ.* August 1988:42-46.

Occupational Safety and Health Administration, Department of Labor. *Hazard Communication Guidelines for Compliance.* Washington, DC: Occupational Safety and Health Administration; 1988. OSHA Document 3111.

O'Neill B, Stone J. Right to Know laws: a guide to maintaining compliance. *Occup Health Saf.* June 1988:28-36,49.

Phifer L, Matthews C. A small quantity approach to laboratory economy and safety. *Am Lab.* August 1978.

Samways M. Functionally illiterate worker also has right-to-understand. *Occup Health Saf.* May 1987:49-53.

Samways M. OSHA voluntary guidelines provide blueprint for employee training. *Occup Health Saf.* May 1987:68-75.

Task Force on Occupational Health and Safety. *Informing Workers of Chemical Hazards: The OSHA Hazard Communication Standard.* Washington, DC: American Chemical Society; 1985.

Chapter 4

The Occupational Exposures to Hazardous Chemicals Standard

4.1 THE LABORATORY STANDARD[1]

The Occupational Safety and Health Administration (OSHA) requires employers to meet the criteria of the ruling "Occupational Exposures to Hazardous Chemicals in Laboratories" (OSHA Standard 1910.1450, commonly referred to as the "Laboratory Standard").[2] The ruling became effective May 1, 1991, with implementation required by January 31, 1991.[1] The contents of this ruling will be discussed elsewhere, but a significant and essential part of this standard is the implementation of a chemical hygiene plan to minimize personnel exposures to hazardous chemicals. The primary goal of this regulation is to educate workers on the proper handling, storage, and disposal of hazardous chemicals rather than to create unnecessary anxiety. It is expected that compliance with this standard will result in a 10% reduction in the incidence of chemical-related illnesses and injuries in the workplace.[2]

These training materials, procedures, and information have been developed to help you understand and comply with the requirements of this standard. Review each category and determine how your current procedures may comply with the requirements of this standard.

Because the standard clearly mandates training in the "specific area" in which the personnel are working, it is necessary that individual sections of the laboratory consider their procedures and develop a chemical hygiene plan for that section. Complete details of the overall institution plan need not be included in this "section-specific plan" but should be readily available in the institution plan, if more detailed explanations of the plan become necessary.

4.1.1 LABORATORY STANDARD COMPLIANCE

The Occupational Exposures to Hazardous Chemicals in Laboratories Standard is frequently referred to as the "Laboratory Standard." It is important to understand that the standard is composed of very specific and defined sections including the "Chemical Hygiene Plan" (Table 4.1). Although frequently the entire standard is referred to as the chemical hygiene

Table 4.1 SIGNIFICANT SECTIONS OF THE LABORATORY STANDARD

The scope and application of the standard

Definitions and terminology used in the standard

Permissible exposure limits

The chemical hygiene plan requirements

Employee information and training requirements

Medical examination and consultations

Hazard identification, labels, and MSDSs

Respirator requirements

Recordkeeping requirements

plan, the plan is but one section. It is necessary to address each of the standard's sections when developing a program for compliance. To make matters somewhat more confusing, the Hazard Communication Standard and the Laboratory Standard frequently overlap in their mandates to provide a comprehensive health and safety program: the Hazard Communication Standard to ensure that workers can protect themselves from hazards associated with chemicals and the Laboratory Standard to implement measures to minimize exposures to hazardous chemicals.

4.1.2   SCOPE AND APPLICATION OF THE STANDARD

4.1.2 A   WHO IS COVERED BY THIS RULING?
All employees engaged in "laboratory use" of hazardous chemicals.

4.1.2 B   COVERAGE DOES NOT APPLY WHEN
The use of chemicals does not provide exposures, such as chemically impregnated media, ie, "dip and read" tests; commercially prepared kits, ie, pregnancy tests in which all reagents are contained in a kit form.

4.1.3   DEFINITIONS OF TERMS USED IN THE STANDARD[2]

The Occupational Exposure to Hazardous Chemicals in Laboratories Standard lists in detail a number of applications and definitions of terms used in the standard. Listed here are those definitions that are considered to be of particular significance for understanding the application of the standard. (A complete list can be found in the standard itself.)

Laboratory: A facility where "laboratory use" of hazardous chemicals occurs on a "laboratory scale."
Laboratory Use: This indicates that multiple chemicals and chemical procedures are used; procedures are not part of a production process; and procedures are on a "laboratory scale."
Laboratory Scale: Working with chemicals for which handling of containers for transfer, reactions, etc, can be safely performed by one person.
Hazardous Chemical: A chemical which shows significant evidence that chronic health effects may occur in exposed employees.
Action Level (AL): A concentration of hazardous chemicals that requires certain activities such as exposure monitoring or medical surveillance.
Permissible Exposure Limits (PELs): An 8-hour time-weighted average of exposure to a substance that should not be exceeded, based on OSHA determinations.

4.1.4   EMPLOYEE EXPOSURE LIMITS

• Initial monitoring (if there is reason to believe that an exposure has occurred)
• Periodic monitoring (if an exposure has occurred)

4.1.5   CHEMICAL HYGIENE PLAN REQUIREMENTS

Develop a plan wherever hazardous chemicals are used in the workplace which protects employees from the health hazards of chemicals, and keeps exposures below specified limits.

Table 4.2 lists the requirements that should be met. Figure 4.1 is an example of a statement of implementation of a chemical hygiene plan.

4.1.5 A   RESPONSIBILITIES OF THE CHEMICAL HYGIENE OFFICER

The chemical hygiene officer works with administration and employees to develop and implement policies and practices; monitors procurement, use, and disposal of chemicals; ensures that the program is audited and maintained; assists managers (supervisors) in developing precautions and adequate facilities; knows current legal regulations; continually seeks ways to improve the program; and reviews and updates the plan as necessary on an annual basis.

Table 4.2   CHEMICAL HYGIENE PLAN REQUIREMENTS

Develop and provide a plan to protect personnel from health hazards of hazardous chemicals.

The plan must be readily available.

Provide specific elements to ensure protection.

Implement standard operating procedures for the use of chemicals.

Identify/implement controls to reduce exposures.

Take specific measures to ensure properly functioning equipment.

Provide personnel information and training.

Provide medical consultation and examinations where applicable.

Provide for prior approval for use of hazard-specific chemicals.

Designate responsible personnel—a chemical hygiene officer.

Provide **protection from** particularly hazardous chemicals.

Review/evaluate effectiveness and update plan annually.

Figure 4.1   STATEMENT OF IMPLEMENTATION OF THE CHEMICAL HYGIENE PLAN

This policy is implemented to protect laboratory workers from health hazards associated with the use of hazardous chemicals in the laboratory. It is designed to identify actual and potential employee exposure, as well as to set forth responsibilities and activities to enhance employee safety. This policy, as well as the OSHA Standard (1910.1450) requiring that this policy be implemented, shall be available to personnel at all times through the chemical hygiene officer.

The Chemical Hygiene Officer for this laboratory facility is _____

Date of Implementation _____

4.1.5 B RESPONSIBILITIES OF MANAGERS AND SUPERVISORS

Managers and supervisors ensure that policies, procedures, and safety precautions are consistently practiced; train and educate employees; and maintain a safe working environment.

4.1.5 C RESPONSIBILITIES OF THE LABORATORY PERSONNEL

Laboratory personnel should develop good personal chemical hygiene habits and consistently adhere to facility policies and safe work practices.

NOTE: It is important that the responsibilities of the Chemical Hygiene Officer, of the managers and supervisors, and of laboratory personnel be included as part of the chemical hygiene plan.

4.1.6 EMPLOYEE INFORMATION AND TRAINING REQUIREMENTS

- Employees must be provided information and training in hazards in their area.
- Training at initial assignment of work and new exposures should be given and refresher training given at the discretion of employer. (Annual retraining is recommended.)
- Employees shall be informed of the contents of the standard; location and availability of the plan; PELs for hazardous chemicals; signs and symptoms associated with exposures; and location and availability of reference materials. Figure 4.2 is a training compliance checklist for employers.
- Training requirements include methods to detect hazardous chemicals; physical and health hazards of chemicals; methods of protection; and applicable details of the plan.
- It is the intent of the laboratory to make available to all personnel as much information and literature as possible regarding the chemicals that they must work with. Personnel are encouraged to request information and use textbooks and reference materials to become as knowledgeable about chemical hazards and the appropriate precautions.

Figure 4.2 TRAINING AND INFORMATION COMPLIANCE CHECKLIST

[ ] Information and training at time of initial work assignment and prior to new exposures

[ ] Frequency of refresher information and training to be determined by employer (annually)

[ ] Textbooks and reference materials available from the chemical hygiene officer

[ ] Written chemical hygiene plan available to all personnel

[ ] OSHA's listing of PELs for regulated substances available to all personnel

[ ] Signs and symptoms associated with exposures available to all personnel

[ ] MSDSs available to all personnel

[ ] Personnel trained in methods used to detect presence or release of hazardous substances

[ ] Personnel trained in physical and health hazards of chemicals used in the laboratory

[ ] Measures employees can take to protect themselves from chemical exposures

[ ] Personnel training in applicable details of the chemical hygiene plan

---

4.1.6 A   TEXTBOOKS AND REFERENCE MATERIALS
Available from the chemical hygiene officer

4.1.6 B   INVENTORY LIST OF CHEMICALS
Maintained and updated regularly

4.1.6 C   OTHER MATERIALS AND INFORMATION
Available from the chemical hygiene officer:
- A written chemical hygiene plan
- OSHA's PELs for regulated substances
- OSHA's Laboratory Standard
- Signs and symptoms associated with exposures
- Material safety data sheets (MSDSs)

4.1.6 D   INITIAL AND ONGOING TRAINING
Is provided, and participation by personnel is required

4.1.6 E   NEW EMPLOYEE ORIENTATION
Training program is required and includes:
- Methods/observations used to detect the presence or release of a hazardous chemical
- Physical and health hazards of chemicals used in the work area
- Measures employees can take to protect themselves from chemical hazards
- Applicable details of the chemical hygiene plan

4.1.6 F   EMPLOYEE TRAINING
- Will be an ongoing part of the chemical hygiene program
- Training shall be provided at the time of an employee's initial assignment of a work area or prior to new exposure assignments.
- Frequency of training shall be determined by the employer; annual review and retraining is strongly recommended.
- Safety training sessions will be documented. Tests may be administered to verify knowledge and understanding of material presented.

4.1.6 G   OBJECTIVES OF THE TRAINING PROGRAM
- Locate the potentially hazardous chemicals in the laboratory.
- Recognize chemical labeling and its meaning.
- Discuss the major components of the facility's standard labeling system.
- Locate the MSDS book in the laboratory.
- Locate the health hazard, physical hazard, environmental protection, and special protection sections of the MSDS and explain their use.
- Identify the laboratory chemical hygiene officer by name and title.
- Identify the appropriate personal protective equipment (PPE) and demonstrate its use.
- Demonstrate emergency procedures in case of a hazardous chemical spill.
- Describe the environmental monitoring protocol.

4.1.7 MEDICAL CONSULTATION AND EXAMINATION

- Provide medical attention when a sign or symptom of exposure develops; when exposure routinely is above the AL; and when an event takes place that results in exposure.
- Is provided by a licensed physician
- Complete exposure information provided to the physician
- Physician's written opinion

4.1.8 HAZARD IDENTIFICATION, LABELS, AND MSDS

Ensure intact labels; MSDSs on all hazardous chemicals; and identification of chemicals produced in the laboratory.

4.1.9 RESPIRATORS

Provide as appropriate. Consult Respiratory Protection Standard (29 CFR 1910.134) for refinements including selection, training, fitting use, and maintenance.

4.1.10 RECORDKEEPING

Any monitoring or medical information on each employee should be kept and transferred as required, for the term of employment plus 30 years.

4.2 A CHEMICAL HYGIENE PLAN[1,2]

4.2.1 STANDARD OPERATING PROCEDURES

- All laboratory personnel shall familiarize themselves with the rules and procedures associated with using chemicals in the laboratory.
- The application of safety rules and safe work practices shall be considered as important as the quality and professionalism of work performance.
- Supervisors at each management level shall be responsible for enforcing safety rules and safe work performance through regular performance evaluations and an application of the standard facility disciplinary policy when infractions occur.
- The chemical hygiene officer shall also be responsible for noting unsafe work practices or safety violations during routine hazard surveillance inspections.

4.2.2 GENERAL HEALTH AND SAFETY REGULATIONS

- No smoking, drinking, or eating is permitted in the laboratory.
- No application of cosmetics or lip balms is permitted in the laboratory.
- No pipetting must be done by mouth.
- All accidents must be reported to the immediate supervisor or chemical hygiene officer regardless of injury severity.
- Always wear appropriate protective gloves when handling biological specimens or hazardous chemicals, and wash hands thoroughly afterwards.

- Inspect gloves and glove boxes before use.
- Flammable liquids in volumes from 1 pint to 2 gallons should be stored in approved safety cans. Less than 1 pint of flammable liquid may be stored on the shelf in its original container. The amount of flammable liquid in working areas should be limited to 2 gallons or 1 day's supply.
- Flammable liquids must be kept away from sources of ignition, such as heat sources, sunlight, and electrical switches.
- Containers of gas must be securely fastened to prevent falling over and kept away from open flames.
- Fire extinguishers must be checked regularly by the maintenance department or designated inspector.
- Always know the exact location of all safety and emergency equipment.
- Aisles, exits, and emergency exits must not be blocked for any reason.
- Report any unusual odors, vapors, or smoke at once to your immediate supervisor or chemical hygiene officer.
- No ethyl ether is to be used or stored in the laboratory without prior permission.
- Always wear chemical splash goggles when pouring chemicals. If a splash of a caustic liquid occurs on skin or in eyes, wash the affected area immediately with copious amounts of water. Emergency showers should be used for large body areas. Eye wash station should be used for all splashes to the eyes.
- No items are to protrude beyond the front of shelf limit.
- Never drink from a laboratory container. Never taste or smell a chemical.
- Learn the uses and potential hazards of all equipment in the laboratory. Use equipment only for its intended purpose.
- All containers must be labeled and dated plainly to identify contents and provide warnings. Original labels on containers shall not be removed or defaced. Never fill a container with a material other than that called for on the label.
- Discard all used needles in sharps containers. Do not recap by hand or break needles.
- Handle all blades and knives with caution and dispose of in sharps containers.
- Exhaust hood must be used for toxic and flammable materials. Keep all such materials away from heat and heating elements.
- Pour strong corrosives by slowly tilting the container and pouring down the slides. Always add acid to water, never water to acid.
- Know the proper disposal method for chemical substances.
- Keep gas cylinders securely chained. Always close the needle valve on a gas cylinder before opening the master valve.
- In the event of injury to an employee or patient, supervisors must fill out the appropriate incident report form as soon after the incident as possible.
- Always check with an MSDS or appropriate technical handbook before ordering or using chemicals and procedures with which you are not familiar.
- When setting up experiments or tests, always inform others working in the area of the chemicals being used and possible hazards involved.
- Strong acids and alkalis are to be stored as near floor level as possible, never above eye level.
- Chemicals that could react with each other are not to be stored together. Acetic acid must always be stored away from nitric acid and sulfuric acid. Become familiar with chemical incompatibilities.
- All reagent bottles should have the caps or stoppers checked after each use for tightness.

- Chemicals capable of producing irritating and dangerous vapors will always be handled under exhaust hoods; wear safety goggles. The sash should be lowered to protect the eyes.
- Check both ends of pipettes for breakage to ensure against injury to fingers and inaccurate delivery from the tip when measuring reagents. Discard chipped or broken pipettes in the sharps container.
- In case of accidents and spills, follow these procedures:

    Eye Contact: Flush eyes with water for at least 15 minutes; seek medical attention.

    Ingestion: Encourage the victim to drink large amounts of water.

    Skin Contact: Promptly flush the affected area with water and remove any contaminated clothing. If symptoms persist, seek medical attention.
- Wash areas of exposed skin well before leaving the laboratory area.
- Practical jokes or other behavior that might confuse, startle, or distract another worker are strictly prohibited.
- During unattended operations such as distillation, leave the lights on, place appropriate signs at doorways, and provide for containment of toxic substances in the event of failure of a utility service such as cooling water.
- A hood or other form of local ventilation should be used when working with any appreciable volatile substance with a threshold limit value (TLV) of less than 50 ppm. Leave the hood on when it is not in active use if toxic substances are in it or if it is uncertain if adequate general laboratory ventilation will be maintained when it is off.

4.2.3   ADDITIONAL PRECAUTIONS

4.2.3 A   EXTRAHAZARDOUS MATERIALS

Due to the unique and added degree of hazard presented by certain chemical classifications, the following additional precautions are also necessary.

- Designated areas will be established when PELs or TLVs are routinely exceeded or exposure may be excessively high. These areas should be identified and labeled as "designated areas."
- Special training should be given to those workers who must enter the area.
- Prior approval (Figure 4.3) from the administrative director of the laboratory or chemical hygiene officer shall be required for any procedure involving any extrahazardous chemical that is not a preestablished routine procedure for which a standard safe operating practice has been established such as allergens and embryotoxics. A list of such procedures is available from the chemical hygiene officer.

4.2.3 B   MODERATE, CHRONIC, OR HIGH ACUTE TOXICITY CHEMICALS

The following precautions must be taken when working with chemicals of moderate, chronic, or high acute toxicity. A complete listing of these chemicals should be available from the chemical hygiene officer.

- Always use a fume hood with a face velocity of at least 60 linear feet per minute.
- A minimum of two people should be present at all times when a compound of high toxicity or unknown toxicity is being handled.
- Skin contact will be avoided through the use of appropriate gloves and long sleeves such as laboratory coats or suitable long gloves or gauntlets.
- Breakable containers of chemicals must be stored in chemically resistant trays.

Figure 4.3 DESIGNATION OF APPROVAL PRIOR TO APPLICATION FOR CHEMICALS AND PROCEDURES

No new chemical, chemical compound, or laboratory procedure may be ordered, handled, or applied without the specific prior, written approval of the administrative director of the laboratory.

Chemicals or procedures that currently require prior approval for use or application include:

Chemical Name (not formula)	Procedure Use	Specific Hazard

Comments/Special Instructions:

All established procedures and use of chemicals and chemical compounds are listed, approved, and annually reviewed in individual laboratory section procedure manuals.

Approved by _____ Title _____ Date _____

_____

- Cover work and storage surfaces in fume hoods in areas where the chemicals are being handled with removable, absorbent, plastic-backed paper.
- Always wash hands and arms immediately after working with these materials.
- The chemical hygiene officer should maintain records of the amounts of these materials on hand, the amounts used, and the names of workers involved.
- When chemical spills occur outside the hood, personnel should immediately evacuate the area and warn others. The laboratory-wide chemical spill response policy will be activated.

NOTE: Specifics for individual chemicals falling into this category are available from the chemical hygiene officer. These sample precautions and additional information are found in *Prudent Practices for Handling Hazardous Chemicals in Laboratories*, published by the National Research Council.[3]

4.2.3 C HIGH-TOXICITY CHEMICALS

The following precautions must be taken when working with chemicals of high chronic toxicity. A complete listing of chemicals is available from the chemical hygiene officer.

- Conduct all transfers and work with these substances in a controlled area or portion of an area designated for use of highly toxic substances.

- Preapproval must be obtained when disposing of these materials.
- Any vacuum pumps used shall be protected from contamination with scrubbers or high-efficiency particulate air (HEPA) filters vented into a hood. All material should be decontaminated before being removed from the controlled area.
- All protective apparel is to be removed and placed in labeled containers on leaving a controlled area.
- Personnel are required to thoroughly wash hands, forearms, face, and neck after working with chemicals in this category.
- A vacuum cleaner equipped with a HEPA filter or a wet mop must be used instead of dry sweeping if the toxic substance is a dry powder and there is an accidental spill.
- Personnel working with substances in this category on a regular basis shall be examined by a medical professional at least on an annual basis.
- The chemical hygiene officer is responsible for maintaining records of substances in this category stored in the laboratory including amounts stored, amounts used, date of use, and the names of users.
- All controlled areas must be conspicuously marked with appropriate warning signs and signs restricting access to the area. All containers of these substances must also be labeled indicating contents and appropriate warnings.

4.2.4 CHEMICAL PROCUREMENT, DISTRIBUTION, AND STORAGE

- All chemicals ordered must have prior approval by the chemical hygiene officer. The procurement, distribution, and storage of chemicals are of vital importance in maintaining a safe laboratory environment.
- All chemicals are to be received in a central location, as designated, before being transported to the laboratory section or storeroom area.
- No chemical container or cylinder of compressed gas must be received in the laboratory without appropriate identification and labeling (ANSIZ-129).
- All dock, storeroom, or other personnel responsible for receiving chemicals must be identified and appropriately trained regarding safe chemical precautions.
- Laboratory personnel receiving supplies are responsible for comparing received chemicals with those on the chemical inventory list and updating the list as necessary.
- Any new chemicals must be noted and the chemical hygiene officer notified in order that an MSDS is obtained prior to or on receiving the chemical.
- The chemical hygiene officer is responsible for controlling access to the stock area.
- Hazardous chemicals should be identified and segregated from other supplies or chemicals.
- Specific exhaust hoods closest to the stock area shall be designated for temporarily storing containers of hazardous substances that may be damaged or are leaking.
- Chemicals classified as highly toxic must be kept in rigid, chemically resistant, secondary containers. Other precautions may be necessary. Consult the chemical hygiene officer.
- Stored chemicals should be examined periodically in conjunction with regular laboratory safety inspections, at least annually.
- The stock area must not be used as a preparation area, repackaging area, or chemical transfer area.
- All flammable liquids must be stored in the flammable liquid storage cabinet. Doors are to be kept closed at all times, metal containers or metal stock shelves are to be grounded. See specific guidelines for flammable liquids.

- The method of transport of chemicals between stock areas and laboratory sections must reflect the potential danger posed by the specific substance. Hand-carried chemicals are to be placed in an outside container or acid carrying bucket. Carts used for transporting chemicals must be stable and have rims to prevent chemicals from falling off and wheels large enough to negotiate uneven surfaces. Small amounts of flammable liquids may only be transported in rugged, pressure-resistant, nonventing containers.

4.2.5   HAZARDOUS CHEMICALS IN THE WORK AREA

- Only minimal working quantities of hazardous chemicals are maintained in the work area.
- All chemical containers are to be labeled appropriately.
- Storage of hazardous chemicals on bench tops or in ventilation hoods shall be considered unacceptable.
- Chemicals must be kept away from heat and out of direct sunlight.
- Chemical incompatibilities should be continuously considered. A table of incompatible chemicals is to be posted on the safety resource bulletin board. (See also 4.5.9 K.)
- Refrigerators should not be used for the storage of chemicals unless they are specifically designated for the appropriate hazard (flammability, explosion-proof lighting, and electrical fixtures).

4.2.6   ENVIRONMENTAL MONITORING

Initial monitoring of employee exposure (to any substance regulated by a standard that requires monitoring) should be conducted. If there is reason to believe that an AL or PEL is routinely exceeded, scheduled regulatory standard–mandated monitoring will be conducted. Due to the small quantities of most chemicals used in the laboratory, regular instrumental monitoring of airborne concentrations is not normally justified. Exposure monitoring for chemicals used in small quantities and infrequently relies on the following precautions.

- Ventilation systems, including hoods, should be checked four times a year to ensure proper function and use; consult the chemical hygiene officer for complete information on all ventilation systems.
- Proper protective clothing to avoid skin contact must be verified.
- Good hygiene and laboratory safety practice by workers must be verified.

Formaldehyde and xylene are chemicals that are used frequently and in large quantities in the laboratory. OSHA's Formaldehyde Standard (1910.1048) and Xylene Standard (1910.1000) must be adhered to.

Annual exposure levels are monitored where the chemicals are used and handled, even if exposure levels remain well below ALs, PELs, short-term exposure levels, or TLVs. Results of exposure monitoring must be posted within 15 days of receiving the results to be communicated to exposed personnel in writing. Any results of exposure monitoring exceeding an AL, PEL, short-term exposure level, or TLV should trigger an exposure evaluation for affected employees. Consult the chemical hygiene officer for more information.

4.2.7   HOUSEKEEPING, MAINTENANCE, AND INSPECTIONS

- General housekeeping is performed by the facility environmental services. Laboratory personnel, however, are responsible for keeping their respective work areas orderly and clean.

- Waste materials must be segregated and disposed of in appropriate receptacles.
- Spilled chemicals must be cleaned up immediately in an approved manner. (See also 4.6.1 and 4.6.2 D.)
- Stairs and hallways must not be used as storage areas at any time.
- Access to exits, emergency equipment, and controls should never be blocked.
- Safety/housekeeping inspections must be conducted on a routine and regular basis (quarterly) and the results of the inspections forwarded to the laboratory director. See the chemical hygiene officer for complete details.
- Safety equipment must be maintained in top condition at all times. Inspections of safety equipment may be held in conjunction with the safety/housekeeping inspections. Consult the chemical hygiene officer for specific instructions.

4.2.8 MEDICAL PROGRAM

Medical surveillance must be conducted in a manner consistent with federal OSHA requirements. Consult the chemical hygiene officer for specific instructions. Personnel exposed to airborne contaminants at or above the AL or PEL must receive regular health monitoring through a medical professional. In the event of overexposure, exposure to a spill or leak, or if an employee develops signs or symptoms associated with a hazardous chemical, the employee shall receive medical consultation and evaluation. This shall include follow-up medical examinations thought to be necessary by the examining physician. Employees who regularly work with or frequently handle hazardous chemicals, although not necessarily overexposed, may consult a qualified physician on an individual basis to determine if a regular schedule of medical surveillance is desirable.

First aid for exposure to toxic substances should be administered through the employee health office or a qualified medical professional, if possible. Personnel, however, should be prepared for emergency situations such as thermal or chemical burns, cuts, and fracture wounds from glass or metal, including possible chemical contamination; skin irritation by chemicals; poisoning by ingestion, inhalation, or skin absorption; asphyxiation—chemical or electrical; and injuries to the eyes from splashed chemicals. Exposure to chemical substances such as formaldehyde may, in some individuals, result in sensitivity to a particular chemical, therefore making it necessary to remove the individual from a particular laboratory area. (See also 5.3.)

4.2.9 PERSONAL PROTECTIVE EQUIPMENT

PPE is the last line of defense against injury. Supervisors are responsible for ensuring proper and consistent use of PPE. Personnel must be conscientiously aware of their surroundings and always select and use appropriate protective equipment when handling hazardous chemicals. Lines of defense may include using proper techniques and methods; being properly trained and indoctrinated; and using engineering controls such as exhaust hoods. The following PPE must be provided as appropriate and its use is required by all personnel:
- Full face shields, safety glasses, and chemical goggles
- Aprons: rubber or designated plastic
- Protective gloves, latex, utility, and mesh
- Cartridge and dust/mist respirators and masks
- Self-contained breathing apparatus (SCBA) where appropriate

The following PPE rules apply to all laboratory personnel:

- Eye protection should always be worn when handling or working with chemicals unless protected by a shield or sash on an exhaust hood. Standard safety glasses are not considered acceptable when working with chemicals. Only chemical splash goggles (acid goggles) or face shields that have splash-proof sides are to be used when protection from chemical splash is needed.
- Full face shields that protect the face and throat should be worn when maximum protection from flying particles and harmful liquids is needed. Safety glasses shall be worn with face shields. (This form of protection may be necessary when working with vacuum systems that create the potential for implosion or when a reaction has potential for a mild explosion.)
- Proper protective gloves and other protective clothing, when necessary, must be worn when there is potential for contact with corrosive or toxic materials or materials of unknown toxicity. Gloves shall be selected on the basis of the materials being handled and the degree of hazard involved. Leather-grip gloves must be used if it is necessary to handle broken glassware or when inserting glass tubes into rubber stoppers. Consult the Bloodborne Pathogen Standard for more information on such procedures that may pose an injury hazard. Insulated gloves shall be used when working with temperature extremes (as with cryogenics). Synthetic materials such as Nomex and Keviar can be used briefly up to 100°C.
- Respirators and SCBAs are primarily designed for use in emergency situations or designated procedures and should not be used by personnel unless properly trained and fit tested to use the apparatus.
- Laboratory coats are intended to prevent contact with dirt and minor chemical splashes or spills. Only designated plastic or rubber aprons shall be utilized when handling, transferring, or otherwise using corrosive or irritating liquids such as hydrochloric acid.
- All PPE must be appropriately stored, cleaned, and cared for on an ongoing basis. Cleaning is especially important after exposure to chemicals. Prior to using any PPE, it should be thoroughly examined and inspected for unusual wear, deterioration, holes, cracks, or other imperfections that could result in failure of the equipment and exposure of an individual.

4.2.10 SAFETY AND EMERGENCY EQUIPMENT

Safety and emergency equipment is provided and all personnel shall know where the following equipment is located and trained on its proper care, use, and function.

- Safety shower
- Emergency eye wash station
- Portable fire extinguishers (various types)
- Fire blanket
- Chemical spill kits
- Mercury spill kits
- Broom, dust pan
- Sharps containers
- Fire alarm system

4.2.11 RECORDKEEPING

The chemical hygiene officer establishes and maintains an accurate record of any personnel monitoring results. Records of any medical consultation or examination, including tests or written opinions, must be maintained by the employee health office or appropriate medical professional. All accidents associated with the handling and use of toxic substance must be thoroughly investigated and documented. Records, reports, and correspondence generated in conjunction with carrying out the chemical hygiene plan must be retained indefinitely. Consult the chemical hygiene officer for complete details.

Records maintained should include:
- Safety/housekeeping inspections
- Preventive maintenance performed on all safety equipment
- Incident and accident reports and follow-up information
- Safety training records
- Fire and other emergency drills
- Exposure monitoring results

4.2.12 SIGNS AND LABELS

Appropriate signs and labels are one of the most significant defenses against illness or injury in the laboratory environment. Personnel must conscientiously observe and obey all precautionary warnings as well as submit, attach, or include signs and labels when they are necessary for the protection of personnel. Emergency phone numbers, internal hospital codes, and home phone numbers for key personnel must be posted. Emergency numbers should be memorized by all personnel.

Chemical containers must not have original labels removed or defaced. Each chemical container must have appropriate hazard warnings. (See also 4.4.) An explanation of the laboratory hazard warning system must be posted in prominent locations in the laboratory. All personnel are to be instructed on the meaning of the hazard warning system used and instructed as to the appropriate precautions to be taken when necessary. Special hazards throughout the laboratory must be clearly identified with symbols and wording in English, including:
- Flammable liquid storage
- Biological waste receptacles
- Areas containing radioactive materials
- Storage areas for strong alkalis or acids
- Location of safety equipment clearly marked and identifiable

4.2.13 SPILLS AND ACCIDENTS

The laboratory participates in a facility-wide internal and external disaster plan. Personnel should be familiar with exits and evacuation routes; participate in both types of plans and appropriate drills; be familiar with alarms and facility codes; and know their responsibilities with regard to these alarms and codes.

Personnel are to be designated from each laboratory section (on each shift) for chemical spill response. Initial training and retraining will be given to these individuals. The procedures to be followed in the event of a chemical splash or injury in the laboratory are listed in Table 4.3. Consult with the chemical hygiene officer for specific details.

4.2.14 PREPARING "SECTION-SPECIFIC" HYGIENE PLANS

Too often technologists become overwhelmed with the prospect of determining a chemical hygiene plan that concerns their area or section of the laboratory. In most instances, their section of the laboratory is but a part of a larger laboratory operation and that larger laboratory operation may be part of a still larger institution, medical school, or university complex. In these instances, there may already be an established institution-wide hygiene plan or document that contains many of the requirements that pertain to the laboratory section. It is not necessary, therefore, that a complete hygiene plan be written but rather a "section-specific" plan that pertains to the hazards of that specific area and a plan that will ultimately become part of the larger document. This fact considerably lightens the responsibility of the technologist who has been asked to represent the department with regard to hazardous materials.

The section-specific chemical hygiene plan sheets presented in Figures 4.4 and 4.5 are examples of how a specific area of the laboratory can identify its hazardous chemicals. Standard operating

Table 4.3 CHEMICAL SPLASH OR INJURY EMERGENCY PROCEDURES*

EYE CONTACT
_____

Immediately flush eyes with water for 15 minutes.

Obtain copy of MSDS for chemical(s) involved.

See health professional for medical evaluation or treatment, if appropriate.

Complete work-related accident or incident form.

SKIN CONTACT
_____

Immediately flush affected area with water, remove any contaminated clothing.

Obtain MSDS for chemical(s) involved.

See health professional for evaluation or treatment, if appropriate.

Complete work-related accident or incident form.

INGESTION
_____

Drink large amounts of water.

Obtain MSDS for chemical(s) involved.

See health professional for evaluation or treatment, if appropriate.

Complete work-related accident or incident form.

* *Federal Register CFR 1910.1450 Appendix A,(E) General Rules for Working with Chemicals (a) Accidents and Spills.*

Figure 4.4 SECTION-SPECIFIC INFORMATION FOR A CHEMICAL HYGIENE PLAN

Laboratory Section _____ Supervisor _____

Average No. of Occupants _____

Significant use of commercially prepared kits   [ ] Yes   [ ] No

Primary function and procedures _____

_____

_____

_____

Significant chemical hazards
(also see attached chemical specific information data)

Chemical   Procedure   Primary Hazard _____

_____

_____

_____

_____

Hazardous chemicals routinely used
(also see attached chemical specific information)

[ ] Carcinogens or suspected carcinogen   [ ] Solvents

[ ] Compressed gas   [ ] Oxidizers

[ ] Flammables   [ ] Reactives

[ ] Dyes   [ ] Radioactive

[ ] Acids   [ ] Other

Comments or exceptions _____

_____

_____

_____

Prepared by (title) _____   Date _____

Date reviewed _____   Verified by _____   Title _____

_____

_____

_____

procedures, essential laboratory safety, and chemical hygiene are covered in the overall laboratory chemical hygiene plan. Therefore, it is necessary that only chemical-specific data with regard to hazardous chemicals in each laboratory section be included in these information sheets. These sheets should include all relevant chemicals used in the area. Additional information concerning specific chemicals or procedures, such as MSDSs or narratives, can be included. Indicate these attachments where appropriate. Do not hesitate to expand or include any additional information that is deemed relevant to the health and safety of personnel.

Sections of the laboratory might include individual chemical hygiene assessments of histology, which could have material specifically for the grossing area, special stains, and immunohistochemistry, cytology, and each section of the clinical laboratory as well. The important thing is to recognize the hazards in each area and identify them in the chemical hygiene plan.

Figure 4.5 SECTION-SPECIFIC INFORMATION

Laboratory Section _____ Supervisor _____

Hazardous chemicals used routinely

Chemical _____ Procedure _____ Primary Hazard _____

_____

_____

_____

_____

_____

_____

_____

_____

_____

_____

_____

_____

_____

Prepared by _____ Date _____

It is appropriate to include in these sheets the name of the supervisor, average number of occupants working in the area, and a brief description of the primary procedures for that section. Separate listings of hazardous chemicals most commonly used are made, and another listing is provided for chemicals that have been identified as significant chemical hazards, such as formaldehyde and xylene. An additional listing can include the chemicals used in the section. It is a good idea to have space for additional comments or exceptions that may be appropriate for that particular section of the laboratory. When completed by each section, these sheets can be placed in the overall laboratory chemical hygiene plan as an indexed appendix. This addition will provide for a completed chemical hygiene plan for the entire facility.

4.3   HAZARDOUS CHEMICALS

4.3.1   WHAT IS A HAZARDOUS CHEMICAL?[4]

A substance is considered to be hazardous if it has one or more of the following characteristics:
- If it is ignitable
- If it is corrosive
- If it is reactive
- If it contains toxic constituents

To be more specific, hazardous chemicals may demonstrate the following characteristics:
- Ignitability, having a flash point of less than 140°F or is subject to spontaneous heating
- Toxicity, if the TLV is below 500 ppm (gas or vapor), below 500 mg/m^3 (fumes), or below 25 mppcf (dust)
- A single lethal dose (LD50) below 500 mg/kg
- If a substance is subject to polymerization with the release of large amounts of energy
- If it is a strong oxidizer or reducer. An oxidizer may react, producing fire or explosion, when exposed to another oxidizer or on coming into contact with an organic compound. Chromic acid and perchloric acid are good examples of such a reaction. A reducer is an agent that removes oxygen from material, as in the Prussian blue reaction between hydrochloric acid and potassium permanganate
- If a substance may cause first degree burns to the skin in a short time of exposure or if it is systemically toxic by skin contact
- If a substance is capable of producing dusts, gases, fumes, vapor, mists, or smoke which has one or more hazardous characteristics

4.3.2   HOW DO YOU KNOW IF A SUBSTANCE IS HAZARDOUS?[4]

4.3.2 A   UNLESS YOU KNOW, CONSIDER IT SO!
Unless you absolutely know that a particular substance is harmless, consider all chemicals to be potentially hazardous and proceed accordingly.

4.3.2 B   CONSULT RESOURCE MATERIALS BEFORE YOU ORDER

Before you order any new substance, consult resource materials to identify any known hazards. Is there an alternative to its use? Order only what you actually need and do not order the substance at all if it cannot be properly handled, used, and disposed of safely.

4.3.2 C   LABELS ON CONTAINERS

Shipping containers provide Department of Transportation and National Fire Protection Agency (NFPA) information. Labels also provide complete information regarding the chemical including:

- Substance name
- Quantity
- Catalog number
- Lot analysis listing impurities
- Precautionary panel, which describes manufacturer's labeling system; principal hazards, signal words for the degree of hazard; rating scale for specific hazards; recommendations for protective equipment; spill control and storage; handling of substance; and first-aid measures

4.3.2 D   MATERIAL SAFETY DATA SHEETS

Required for all hazardous chemicals in the laboratory, these data sheets must be kept on file and available to all personnel. Information should include:

- Identity of the chemical
- Physical and chemical characteristics
- Known acute and chronic health effects
- Exposure limits
- Whether substance is carcinogenic or not
- Precautionary measures
- Emergency and first-aid procedures
- Identification of organization that is responsible for preparing the MSDS

4.3.3   TARGET ORGAN EFFECTS OF CHEMICALS[5]

The following list of target organ effects should be posted in a central location for access by all personnel.

4.3.3 A   BLOOD AND HEMATOPOIETIC SYSTEM

Decreases hemoglobin function; deprives body of oxygen
> *Signs and Symptoms:* Cyanosis, loss of consciousness
> *Chemicals:* Carbon monoxides, cyanides

4.3.3 B   CUTANEOUS HAZARDS

Chemicals that affect the dermal layer of the skin
> *Signs and Symptoms:* Defatting of the skin, rashes, irritation
> *Chemicals:* Ketones, chlorinated compounds

4.3.3 C   EYE HAZARDS
Chemicals that affect the eye or visual capacity
> *Signs and Symptoms:* Conjunctivitis, corneal damage
> *Chemicals:* Organic solvents, acids, formalin

4.3.3 D   HEPATOTOXINS
Chemicals that produce liver damage
> *Signs and Symptoms:* Jaundice, liver enlargement
> *Chemicals:* Carbon tetrachloride, uranium

4.3.3 E   NEPHROTOXINS
Chemicals that produce kidney damage
> *Signs and Symptoms*: Edema, proteinuria
> *Chemicals:* Halogenated hydrocarbons, uranium

4.3.3 F   NEUROTOXINS
Chemicals that produce their primary toxic effects on the nervous system
> *Signs and Symptoms:* Narcosis, behavioral changes, decrease in motor function
> *Chemicals:* Mercury, carbon disulfide, xylene, mercuric chloride

4.3.3 G   LUNG DAMAGE
Chemicals that irritate or damage pulmonary tissue
> *Signs and Symptoms:* Cough, tightness in chest, shortness of breath
> *Chemicals:* Silica, asbestos

4.3.3 H   REPRODUCTIVE TOXINS
Chemicals that affect the reproductive capabilities including chromosomal damage (mutations) and effects on fetuses (teratogenesis)
> *Signs and Symptoms:* Birth defects, sterility
> *Chemicals:* Lead

4.3.4   SIGNIFICANT TYPES OF CHEMICAL HAZARDS[1]

4.3.4 A   SPECIFIC HAZARDOUS CHEMICAL CONTROL INFORMATION
It should be remembered that adequate ventilation is essential when handling any chemical. Certain of the following types of chemicals are frequently used in laboratories (Table 4.4).

4.3.4 B   FORMALDEHYDE
The OSHA Formaldehyde Standard as published in the *Federal Register* (December 3, 1987, Vol. 52, No. 233) and current revisions (1993) lists more detailed instructions.

Formaldehyde is used in two forms: 37% (full strength) solution and 10% (4% working solution) formalin. Formaldehyde is considered hazardous as an irritant, sensitizer, and potential human carcinogen. Personnel handling formaldehyde during any laboratory procedure, such as grossing tissue, specimen preparation, and processing tissue, are required to wear PPE: gloves, safety goggles, and laboratory coat with apron, if appropriate. A well-ventilated area is essential. Monitoring of formaldehyde levels is covered in the Formaldehyde Standard.

If a formaldehyde spill occurs:
• Proceed as instructed in 4.6.1 A.
• Cleanup personnel must wear a full-face respirator, protective clothing, and goggles, if appropriate, with respirator.
• Cleanup materials must be carefully bagged and disposed of in an appropriate manner.

4.3.4 C   ALCOHOLS

Ethyl alcohol is commonly used in processing and staining specimens in both cytology and histology sections of the laboratory. It is hazardous because it is highly flammable and is toxic. Methyl alcohol is highly poisonous. Personnel handling alcohols should wear protective gloves, safety glasses, and laboratory coats when pouring material from containers or any procedure in which splashes can reasonably be anticipated. All work should be performed in a well-ventilated area.

Alcohols may be discarded into the sink drain with copious amounts of water to eliminate the risk of flammability or toxicity. However, recycling of waste alcohols is highly cost-effective and environmentally sound. It must be understood that continually changing regulations—federal and state and even local ordinances— may not permit the discharge of alcohols into drain systems. When establishing your procedures, it is important to check existing regulations that may have an impact on your facility.

If an alcohol spill occurs proceed as instructed in 4.6.1 A. After evaporation under a hood, waste materials may be placed and disposed of in the usual manner.

4.3.4 D   XYLENE AND XYLENE SUBSTITUTES

Xylene and xylene substitutes are also commonly used in processing tissue and staining both histology and cytology specimens. Although not officially recognized as a carcinogen, xylene is treated as one in most laboratories. (NIOSH Bulletin No. 48 raises the question of whether xylene is a neurotoxin.) Xylene is also highly flammable and is a skin irritant in some individuals.

Table 4.4   CHEMICALS FREQUENTLY USED IN LABORATORIES

Fixatives such as formaldehyde

Alcohols

Solvents such as xylene

Acids

Bases

Carcinogens

Xylene is an organic chemical (not water soluble), and it can be absorbed directly through the skin into the blood system. For this reason, a xylene substitute may be used, wherever appropriate, and is for the most part considered to be substantially less toxic than xylene. However, because these substitutes are not without hazardous effects, they should be handled and disposed of appropriately. Some substitutes may contain limonene, which is an irritant and sensitizer and therefore must be handled with appropriate precautions.

Personnel handling xylene and xylene substitutes must wear protective gloves, safety glasses, and laboratory coats. A well-ventilated workstation is essential.

Xylene waste is collected in waste containers (with appropriate warning labels) for disposal by a licensed transporter. It may NOT be poured down sink drains. However, recycling waste xylene and xylene substitutes is an environmentally sound and more cost-effective practice. Distillation techniques for recycling have proven to be highly effective in reclaiming these solvents and require a minimum of operator time.

If a xylene or xylene substitute spill occurs proceed as directed in 4.6.1 A. Place contaminated materials under a hood until complete evaporation has occurred, and then dispose of in sealed or tied bags.

4.3.4 E   ACIDS
Acids are chemicals having a pH value less than 7.0 (hydrochloric, sulfuric, and acetic acids). The lower the pH, the stronger the acid and the greater the hazard!

Personnel working with acids must wear protective gloves, safety glasses, and protective laboratory coats/aprons because acids are extremely caustic and burn tissue on contact. Remember that when opening an acid bottle, fumes combine with water vapor in the air to make an "acid cloud." Breathing this cloud could result in serious injury or death and must be avoided. Acid spills are particularly dangerous because of this cloud.

Where possible, acids are stored in a specially labeled "acid cabinet" located at floor level. Never store acids above eye level. In the event of an accident, this practice may prevent unnecessary blindness. Acids must be handled only in a ventilated hood.

If an acid spill occurs:
• Notify the appropriate personnel of the spill, apply absorbent if possible, and evacuate the area immediately.
• For large spills, cleanup must be done by personnel wearing appropriate protective equipment (rubber suit with respirator). Acids attack both skin and clothing.
• The spill must be neutralized with sodium bicarbonate. Remove absorbent to ventilated hood for evaporation and discard after bagging disposal materials securely. (See also 4.3.5 F.)

4.3.4 F   BASES

Bases are chemicals having a pH value greater than 7.0 (ammonium hydroxide and potassium hydroxide). The higher the pH, the stronger the base!

Bases are extremely hazardous because they are caustic—they dissolve tissue. It is essential that acids be stored separately from bases. Contact between the two chemicals can result in explosion.

Bases must be handled with gloves, safety goggles, and protective clothing. They must be used under a hood. Inhalation of vapors from an opened bottle can cause unconsciousness or death.

If a base spill occurs:
- Use protective clothing as with acids.
- Contain with absorbent.
- Neutralize with weak citric acid.
- Remove to ventilated hood, evaporate, bag, and discard.

4.3.4 G   CARCINOGENS

Essentially all chemical dyes and heavy metals (toxic) found in the laboratory should be considered at least potential carcinogens. Because information is lacking on the nature of many of these agents, it is prudent to treat all chemical dyes and heavy metals with extreme respect unless unequivocal data are obtained.

Carcinogens are chemicals that have been proven to cause cancer. If described as a "possible carcinogen," consider it so and treat as a known carcinogen. Carcinogens must be handled in a ventilated hood using protective gloves, safety goggles, and appropriate protective clothing. Carcinogens must not be disposed of into the environment untreated.

4.3.5   HAZARDOUS CHEMICALS IN HISTOLOGY[1,6]

There are several specific categories of chemicals in the laboratory that require specific attention: fixatives, metals (salts and acids), dyes, explosive agents, and others.

4.3.5 A   FIXATIVES

Fixatives are of particular interest in light of the OSHA Formaldehyde Standard. There are several fixatives that require our attention in the histology laboratory.

Formaldehyde: Most common in histology laboratories, formaldehyde irritates the skin and mucous membranes, hardens or "tans" the skin, and causes skin cracking and ulceration. In addition, it may cause blindness or conjunctivitis if the eyes are exposed. Further, it may cause laryngitis, bronchitis, or pneumonia if inhaled. It is a known sensitizer and may be carcinogenic as well.

NOTE: Bis-chloromethyl ether is formed by the reactions of hydrochloric acid and formaldehyde. This chemical induces lung cancer in humans. Certain decalcification procedures, staining procedures, or reactive solutions within a common sink may produce this reaction.

Phenol: A very dangerous chemical. The vapor causes irritation to eyes and mucous membranes. Phenol anesthetizes fingers and whitens skin. Burns may occur on excessive contact. Absorption through the skin causes headaches, dizziness, damage to the kidneys and liver, and possibly dermatitis.

Picric Acid (Alcoholic Fixative Solution): A class A explosive that causes dermatitis. Prolonged exposure may result in skin eruptions, headache, vomiting, and diarrhea. Picric acid is a class A explosive and is readily detonated when dry. It is explosive in greater than 50% solution with water. It forms heat and friction or impact-sensitive salts with many metals such as lead, mercury, copper, or zinc. (See also 4.3.5 E and 4.6.5.)

Potassium Dichromate: As a fixative, it irritates the eyes and respiratory tract; chronic exposure can cause skin ulceration as well as liver and kidney disease. It is carcinogenic and reacts explosively with hydroxylamine.

B-5 Fixative: This popular fixative contains mercuric chloride. It is a poison and chronic exposure can lead to severe nervous system and kidney damage. It is also considered to be carcinogenic.

4.3.5 B   SOLVENTS

Solvents are another important category of chemicals because of their widespread use in histology procedures. Remember, a 1-gallon spill or a reagent chemical results in a surface area of 20 square feet!

Acetone: Highly damaging to the eyes. Highly flammable, reacts violently with chloroform and a base.

Aniline: The solvent base for many dyes, it is a suspected carcinogen. Toxic, with skin contact being the most common entry route.

Benzene: A carcinogen, it attacks the bone marrow and causes leukemia. It also attacks the brain and central nervous system. It is highly flammable. It may explode in combination with oxidants.

Ether: Highly flammable and forms explosive peroxides on exposure to air and light. It should be treated with the greatest respect. A 1% concentration is sufficient to cause an explosion or fire! Store in a cool area in an electrically grounded container or explosion-proof refrigerator.

Glycerol : Produces violent or explosive reactions with oxidizing agents.

Methanol: A poison by inhalation or ingestion. Highly flammable.

Pyridine: Highly flammable. Causes headaches, nausea, and vomiting. Noxious odor.

Toluene: Very flammable. May cause dermatitis, and repeated exposure may produce blood disease.

Xylene: Very flammable. Prolonged exposure can cause dermatitis. May cause headaches, dizziness, nausea, and vomiting. Considered to be a neurotoxin and may cause severe nervous system damage.

4.3.5 C   METALS

Metals (their salts and acids) are a particularly dangerous category of chemicals. Safe use of these chemicals is essential.

Chromic Acid (Chromium Trioxide): It is an irritant and chronic exposure can cause skin ulceration. It is explosive with acetic acid and may ignite acetone, glycerol, methanol, ethanol, and pyridine.

Lead Acetate: May cause central nervous system damage. A carcinogen.

Potassium Permanganate: It is explosive when combined with acetic, hydrochloric, or sulfuric acids, and is flammable when combined with glycerol and solid potassium.

Silver Nitrate: Causes skin pigmentation or burns. May explode when combined with ethanol or charcoal.

Uranyl Acetate: Radioactive, irritates lungs, accumulates uranium in the kidneys causing damage.

4.3.5 D   DYES

Dyes frequently used in histology procedures are frequently overlooked with regard to their safe use. Considering that potential hazards in a large number of these dyes are unknown at this time and certain dyes have been identified as carcinogens or suspected carcinogens, it is vital that their proper use and handling be observed. A good practice when working with dyes, or any chemical for that matter, is simply to consider all of them to be potentially hazardous. Use of a particle mask to prevent inhalation of airborne particles is suggested when an appropriate fume hood is not available. Nonporous gloves, except latex, are recommended when handling dyes. Dyes and certain solvent-based stains penetrate latex material rather quickly.[7] Table 4.5 lists the common dyes used in laboratories and their hazards. Figure 4.6 is a list of common histologic dyes used in laboratories.

4.3.5 E   EXPLOSIVES

Explosives are also a very serious danger in the laboratory. A number of potentially explosive chemicals have already been discussed, such as benzene, ether, glycerol, methanol, chromic acid, potassium dichromate, potassium permanganate, and silver nitrate. Also included in this very important category are the following:

Hydrogen Peroxide: This is a highly dangerous chemical because when heated, shocked, or contaminated, the concentrated material can explode or start fires.

Nitrocellulose (Celloidin, Collodion): Highly explosive when dry. Highly flammable.

Perchloric acid: Like acids, can cause burns. It is potentially explosive in concentrations above 70%.

NOTE: Spillage, which builds up concentrations, must be avoided. Reacts violently with acetic acid, alcohols, formaldehyde, dehydrants, ether, glycerols, and iodides.

Picric Acid: This is a stronger explosive than trinitrotoluene (TNT) and the salts of the acid are even more sensitive explosives. It must be kept out of contact with metals. Never use picric acid near an open flame. Shock will explode it. The acid is received from the manufacturer in a 10% water solution that looks like wet sand. In its wet form it is less dangerous; you must not let the acid become dry. If this happens by evaporation, add distilled water drop by drop, until the crystals appear moist again. (See also 4.3.5 A and 4.6.5.)

Table 4.5   POTENTIAL HAZARDS OF DYES[7]

DYE	HAZARD
Acridine dyes:(quinacrine mustard, quinacrine, arcidine orange, acriflavine hypochloride)	May be mutagenic, and are suspected carcinogens.
Aminoethylcarbazole (AEC)	Carcinogen, treating waste with bleach not recommended
Auramine O (basic yellow 2)	Suspected carcinogen
Brilliant blue	Considered toxic, poisonous
Basic fuchsin	Moderately toxic, potentially explosive
Biebrich scarlet	Considered to be carcinogenic
Fast green FCF	May be carcinogenic.
Crystal violet (Gentian violet)	Carcinogenic, a poison, irritant, potentially explosive, special care needed when handling because easily airborne
Diaminobenzidine (DAB)	A chromagen frequently used in immunohistochemistry. It is a carcinogen. Alternative reagents are frequently substituted for DAB, such as benzidine dihydrochloride, tetramethoxyl benzidine, and paraphenylenediamine, but these chemicals are not without significant hazardous properties also. Treating waste using bleach is not recommended.
Eosin Y	Insufficient data for carcinogenic determination, treat with bleach until solution pale yellow. Neutralize with sodium bicarbonate for drain disposal (if approved).
Gold chloride	It is corrosive.
Hematoxylin	Suspected carcinogen, treat with sodium iodate until brown, neutralize with sodium bicarbonate, drain disposal if approved. Do not use bleach for disposal treatment (toxic chlorine fumes may be produced). Solutions containing mercury are never drain-disposable without removing mercury.
Light green yellowish	May be carcinogenic, inconclusive evidence.
Metanil yellow	May produce reproductive problems.
Methylene blue	Severe eye irritant
Methyl green	Irritant that emits toxic fumes under fire conditions
Pyronin Y	Irritant to eyes, skin, and mucous membranes
Rhodamine B	May be carcinogenic, inconclusive data.
Sudan IV	May be carcinogenic, inconclusive data.
Tartrazine	Ingestion may result in paresthesia.
Toluidine blue O	Blood and gastrointestinal disorder reports

Strong acids, such as hydrochloric, sulfuric, nitric, glacial acetic, and formic acids, have very specific guidelines for use and handling. Failure to follow these instructions may be disastrous. Follow the manufacturers' guidelines for use.

Remember, organic acids such as acetic, formic, and citric acid must be stored separately from strong oxidizing agents such as sulfuric and nitric acids to prevent the interaction of their fumes and resulting corrosion of storage cabinets.

If possible, never receive or use acid containers that are more than 1 quart in size. (Some procedures or facilities may, however, find it necessary to order larger quantities for their needs.)

Never carry acid (or any other reagent) bottle containers by the ring on the side of the bottle top. The ring is for stabilization when pouring only and the ring could come loose like the handle on an old coffee cup.

Never add water to strong acids. Remember, A to W (acid to water). These solutions can produce extreme heat and should be treated appropriately.

Never heat strong acids. For example, heated hydrochloric acid gives off strong chloride fumes which corrode the lungs, cause edema, and can be deadly. (See also 4.3.4 E.)

4.4 CHEMICAL LABELING REQUIREMENTS[1]

The Hazard Communication Standard (HazCom), Occupational Exposure to Hazardous Chemicals in Laboratories Standard (the Laboratory Standard), the Formaldehyde Standard, and the Bloodborne Pathogen Standard all contain instructions for chemical or specimen labeling. Perhaps because of some overlapping of the standards, there is confusion concerning labeling requirements, especially where chemicals are concerned.

Figure 4.6 COMMON HISTOLOGIC DYES – HAZARDOUS PROPERTIES NOT ESTABLISHED

Acid fuchsin	Alcian blue	Alizarian red	Aniline blue
Azocarmine	Azure A, B, C	Bismark brown	Carmine
Chromotrope	Congo Corinth G	Darrow red	Eosin B (not Y)
Ethyl eosin	Gallocyanine	Janus green	Malachite green
Martius yellow	Methylene violet	Methyl green	Methyl orange
Neutral red	Nigrosin	Nile blue	Thionin
Nuclear fast red (Kernechtrot)	Pyronine B, Y	Safranin O	Sudan black B

The NFPA classification "diamond" is not a requirement on chemical labels in the laboratory environment. The NFPA booklet (NFPA 704, *Standard Systems for the Identification of the Fire Hazards of Materials*, 1990) clearly states the following:

1-1 Scope: 1-1.1 This standard (NFPA) shall address the health, flammability, reactivity, and related hazards that may be presented by short-term, acute exposure to a material during handling under conditions of fire, spill, or similar emergencies.

1-2.3: This standard is not applicable to chronic exposure or to nonemergency exposure.

1-3 Purpose: This system is intended to provide basic information to fire fighting, emergency, and other personnel, enabling them to more easily decide whether to evacuate the area or to commence emergency control procedures. It is also intended to provide them with information to assist in selecting fire fighting tactics and emergency procedures.

The NFPA is therefore not appropriate for indicating hazards associated with everyday chemical use. There are, however, hazard identification system designs that resemble the NFPA diamond, while other systems are "bar- or color-coded" in design. Manufacturers must label containers of hazardous chemicals with the following information:
- Identity of the hazardous chemical
- Appropriate hazard warnings
- Name and address of the chemical manufacturer
- Emergency phone numbers

In-house laboratory chemicals that are not in their original containers must be labeled with the following information:
- Identity of the hazardous chemical
- Route of entry to the body
- Health hazard
- Physical hazard
- Target organ affected

The College of American Pathologists publication *Guidelines for Laboratory Safety* (1989) states that "containers of hazardous chemicals must be labeled, tagged, or marked with appropriate hazard warnings including any words, pictures, symbols, or combinations which convey the health and/or physical hazards of the container's contents. Hazard warning must be specific as to the effect of the chemical and specific target organs involved." Furthermore, "Any secondary container into which hazardous chemicals are transferred from labeled containers must also be labeled with the chemical identity of the contents, and any precautionary handling hazards, including specific effects of the chemical and target organs affected. The only permissible exceptions to this requirement are containers intended for immediate use only by the person who does the transfer, and only within the work shift in which the transfer was made."

Also of importance is the following, as stated in the Laboratory Standard: "Therefore, the requirements of OSHA's Hazard Communication Standard concerning the retention of labels accompanying incoming shipments of hazardous chemicals have been incorporated into this standard (Laboratory Standard)." To avoid any confusion that could arise regarding hazard identification relating to the Hazard Communication Standard as distinct from that relating to this standard (Laboratory Standard), OSHA has added three clarifying statements regarding laboratory-generated chemical substances.

- If a chemical substance whose chemical composition is known is produced in the laboratory for its own exclusive use, OSHA requires that available hazard information be provided to the employees who may be exposed to the substance (Figure 4.7). MSDSs and label preparations as required under the Hazard Communication Standard do not apply because under the Laboratory Standard, the laboratory use and laboratory scale definitions are in effect.
- Employers who produce a chemical by-product whose composition is unknown shall make the assumption that the substance is hazardous and require that it be handled according to the chemical hygiene plan.
- The Laboratory Standard clarifies the employer's responsibility where a chemical is produced in the laboratory and shipped to another user outside the laboratory.

4.4.1 COLOR-CODED HAZARD WARNING SYSTEMS (NFPA-TYPE WARNINGS)[8]

Although a number of hazard warning systems are available from commercial sources, all of these color-coded systems are based on NFPA information and are described as NFPA-type systems. Determination of the hazard is listed by color indication as well as a descriptive number identification.

4.4.1 A HEALTH HAZARDS (BLUE)
- 4 Can cause death or major injury despite medical treatment.
- 3 Can cause serious injury despite medical treatment.
- 2 Can cause injury. Requires prompt treatment.
- 1 Can cause irritation if not treated.
- 0 No hazard

4.4.1 B FLAMMABILITY (RED)
- 4 Very flammable gases or very volatile flammable liquid
- 3 Can be ignited at all normal temperatures.
- 2 Ignites if moderately heated.
- 1 Ignites after considerable preheating.
- 0 Will not burn.

Figure 4.7 AN EXAMPLE OF APPROVED LABELING

Acetic Acid

Route of entry: Eyes, skin, nose

Health hazard: Corrosive

Physical hazard: Poison

Target organ: Skin and lungs

4.4.1 C   REACTIVITY (STABILITY) (YELLOW)

- 4   Readily detonates or explodes.
- 3   Can detonate or explode but requires strong initiating force or heating under confinement.
- 2   Normally unstable but will not detonate.
- 1   Normally stable. Unstable at high temperature and pressure. Reacts with water.
- 0   Normally stable. Not reactive with water

4.4.1 D   SPECIAL NOTICE AREA (WHITE)

- POL—Polymerizes under normal conditions.
- W—Water reactive

Table 4.6   HEALTH CODES*

HEALTH CODE	HEALTH EFFECTS
1	Cancer—currently regulated by OSHA as a carcinogen
2	Chronic (cumulative) toxicity—Known or suspected animal or human carcinogen, mutagen (except code 1 chemicals)
3	Chronic (cumulative) toxicity—Long-term organ toxicity other than nervous, respiratory, hematologic, or reproductive
4	Acute toxicity—Short-term high-risk effects
5	Reproductive hazard—Teratogenesis or other reproductive impairment
6	Nervous system disturbances—Cholinesterase inhibition
7	Nervous system disturbances—Effects other than narcosis
8	Nervous system disturbances—Narcosis
9	Respiratory effects other than irritation—Respiratory sensitization, asthmas
10	Respiratory effects other than irritation—Cumulative lung damage
11	Respiratory effects other than irritation—Acute lung damage/edema or other
12	Hematologic (blood) disturbances—Anemias
13	Hematologic (blood) disturbances—Methemoglobinemia
14	Irritation, eyes, nose, throat, skin—Marked
15	Irritation, eyes, nose, throat, skin—Moderate
16	Irritation, eyes, nose, throat, skin—Mild
17	Asphyxiants, anoxiants
18	Explosive, flammable, safety (no adverse effects encountered when good housekeeping practices are followed)
19	Generally low-risk health effects—Nuisance particulates, vapors, gases
20	Generally low-risk health effects—Odor

Adapted from the OSHA Instruction CPL2-2.20A Office of Health Compliance Assistance.[5]

- OXY—Oxidizing agent
- EXP—Explosive heat or shock sensitive
- Radiation symbol—Radiation hazard

4.4.2 CHEMICAL INFORMATION

The health codes listed in Table 4.6 describe the toxicologic properties of the chemical substance.[5] The health code may be used where appropriate, such as in a chemical inventory listing, to indicate a specific chemical hazard.

4.5 CHEMICAL STORAGE[1]

4.5.1 STORE AWAY FROM WATER

The following chemicals react rapidly to water-forming flammable gases, sometimes in explosive concentrations: calcium carbide, potassium metal (store in petroleum), and sodium metal (store in petroleum).

4.5.2 FLAMMABLE OR COMBUSTIBLE

Store the chemicals listed in Table 4.7 in a cool place away from sparks, such as in a ventilated cabinet or open shelf where concentrations of vapor cannot build up.

4.5.3 RAPIDLY POISONOUS

The chemicals listed in Table 4.8 become rapidly poisonous when taken internally, when vapors are inhaled in large concentrations, and when continuous contact with the skin is permitted.

4.5.4 HIGH-RISK GROUP

Particular attention should be given to the hazardous properties of the chemicals listed in Table 4.9. Although mentioned in other categories, they are repeated for emphasis.

4.5.5 STRONG ACIDS

The acids listed in Table 4.10 should be stored away from alkalis in metal cabinets, and drip trays (polyethylene) used.

4.5.6 STRONG ALKALIS

Store the following away from acids: ammonium hydroxide, calcium hydroxide, calcium fluoride (highly corrosive), potassium hydroxide, and sodium hydroxide.

Table 4.7 FLAMMABLE OR COMBUSTIBLE CHEMICALS

Acetone	Hydrocyanic acid
Benzene	Methyl alcohol
Calcium metal, finely divided	Magnesium metal
Carbon disulfide	Red amorphous phosphorus
Ethyl alcohol	Sulfur
Ethyl ether	Xylene
Glacial acetic acid	Yellow phosphorus

Table 4.8 RAPIDLY POISONOUS CHEMICALS

Arsenous trioxide	Barium chloride	Bromine
Carbon disulfide	Copper sulfate	Hydrocyanic acid
Lead acetate	Lead carbonate	Lead nitrate
Magnesium sulfate	Mercuric chloride	Mercuric nitrate
Mercuric oxide	Mercurous chloride	Mercurous nitrate
Metallic mercury	Oxalic acid	Phosphorus
Potassium ferricyanide	Potassium ferrocyanide	Potassium permanganate
Potassium thiocyanate	Sodium oxalate	

Table 4.9 HIGH-RISK CHEMICALS

Benzene	Carbon disulfide
Chlorosulfonic acid	Ethyl ether
Hydrocyanic acid	Hydrofluoric acid
Perchloric acid	Potassium chlorate
Potassium ferricyanide	Potassium ferrocyanide
Potassium metal	Sodium metal
Sodium nitrate	Yellow phosphorus

4.5.7 CHEMICALS THAT IRRITATE, BURN, OR SENSITIZE SKIN AND EYES

Prevent body contact with the following chemicals or remove at once: antimonous trichloride, glass wool, potassium dichromate, powdered antimony metal, silver nitrate, sodium sulfide, sulfinic acid, and zinc chloride.

4.5.8 STRONG OXIDIZING AGENTS

The chemicals listed in Table 4.11 may explode spontaneously if allowed to contact combustible matter.

4.5.9 SPECIFIC CATEGORIES FOR CHEMICAL STORAGE

4.5.9 A FLAMMABLES
- Store in approved safety cans or cabinets that must be grounded and bonded when used.
- Keep away from oxidizing acids and oxidizers.

Table 4.10 STRONG ACIDS

Chlorosulfonic acid	Nitric acid
Formic acid	Perchloric acid
Glacial acetic acid	Phosphoric acid
Hydrochloric acid	Sulfuric acid
Hydrofluoric acid	

Table 4.11 STRONG OXIDIZING AGENTS

Ammonium nitrate	Nickel nitrate
Bromine	Nitric acid
Calcium hypochlorite	Potassium chloride
Chlorine dioxide	Potassium dichromate
Chlorosulfonic acid	Potassium nitrate
Cobaltous nitrate	Potassium permanganate
Hydrogen peroxide	Sodium peroxide (keep dry)
Iodine	Strontium nitrate

- Avoid source of ignition.
- Keep highly volatile flammables in a specially equipped refrigerator.
- Keep fire fighting equipment and spill cleanup materials readily available. Tables 4.12, 4.13, and 4.14 list the liquids, gases, and solids that fall into this category.

4.5.9 B   ACIDS
- Always store below counter level or in acid cabinets.
- Always use bottle carriers for transporting acids.
- Keep away from flammable and combustible materials.
- Keep oxidizing acids away from organic acids (Table 4.15).
- Keep away from bases and active metals such as sodium, potassium, and magnesium.
- Keep away from chemicals that are capable of generating toxic gases on contact such as sodium cyanide and iron sulfide.
- Keep spill kits readily available in case of spills. Figure 4.8 highlights some of the special instructions to be followed when storing acids. (See also 4.3.4 E and 4.3.5 F.)

4.5.9 C   PYROPHORIC CHEMICALS
Table 4.16 lists some pyrophoric chemicals.

4.5.9 D   BASES
- Keep away from acids.
- Inorganic hydroxides must be stored in polyethylene containers.
- Keep spill cleanup materials readily available. Table 4.17 lists some commonly used bases. (See also 4.3.4 F.)

4.5.9 E   LIGHT-SENSITIVE CHEMICALS (TABLE 4.18)
- Avoid exposure to light.
- Store in amber bottles in cool, dry place.

4.5.9 F   PEROXIDE-FORMING CHEMICALS (TABLE 4.19)
- Store in airtight containers in dark, cool, dry place.
- Dispose of before expected date of first peroxide formation.
- Test for presence of peroxides regularly.

CAUTION: **Under proper conditions, these chemicals will form explosive peroxides that can be detonated by shock or heat!**
NOTE: Potassium peroxide exists in the crust around a chunk of potassium. When cut, the peroxide rapidly oxidizes the residual potassium resulting in an explosion!

4.5.9 G   WATER-REACTIVE CHEMICALS
These chemicals react with water to cause flammable or toxic gases or other hazardous conditions. Keep away from water. Store in dry, cool place. Table 4.20 lists the solid and liquid chemicals that fall in this category.

Table 4.12　Flammable Liquids

Acetaldehyde	Ethylamine	Methyl formate
Acetone	Ethyl benzene	Methyl isoburyl ketone
Acetyl chloride	Ethylene dichloride	Methyl methacrylate
Allyl alcohol	Ethyl ether	Methyl propyl ketone
Allyl chloride	Ethyl formate	Morpholine
N-amyl acetate	Furan	Naphtha
N-amyl alcohol	Gasoline	Nitromethane
Benzine	Heptane	Octane
N-butyl acetate	Hexane	Piperidine
N-butyl alcohol	Hydrazine	Propanol
N-butylamine	Isobutyl alcohol	Propyl acetate
Carbon disulfide	Isopropyl acetate	Propylene oxide
Chlorobenzene	Isopropyl ether	Pyridine
Cyclohexane	Mesityl oxide	Styrene
Diethylamine	Methanol	Tetrahydrofuran
Diethyl carbonate	Methyl acetate	Toluene
p-Dioxane	Methyl acrylate	Turpentine
Ethanol	Methylal	Xylene
Ethyl Acetate	Methyl butyl ketone	
Ethyl acrylate	Methyl ethyl ketone	

Table 4.13　Flammable Gases

Acetylene	Ethyl chloride	Hydrogen sulfide
Ammonia	Ethylene	Methane
Butane	Ethylene oxide	Propane
Carbon monoxide	Formaldehyde	Propylene
Ethane	Hydrogen	

Table 4.14　Flammable Solids

Benzoyl peroxide	Phosphorus, yellow
Calcium carbide	Picric acid

Table 4.15 ACID CATEGORIES TO BE STORED SEPARATELY

OXIDIZING ACIDS	ORGANIC ACIDS	OTHER ACIDS
Chromic acid	Acetic acid	Hydrobromous acid
Hydrobromic acid	Benzoic acid	Hydrochloric acid
Iodic acid	Chloroacetic acid	Hydrochlorous acid
Nitric acid	Phenol	Hydrofluoric acid
Perchloric acid	Propionic acid	Hydriodic acid
Sulfuric acid	Sulfamic acid	Nitrous acid
		Phosphoric acid
		Phosphorous acid
		Sulfurous acid

Table 4.16 PYROPHORIC CHEMICALS

Boron

Cadmium*

Calcium*

Chromium*

Diborane

Dichloroborane

2-Furaldehyde

Iron*

Lead*

Manganese*

Nickel*

Phosphorus, yellow (should be stored and cut under water)

Titanium*

Zinc*

* Chemicals that must be stored in a cool, dry place. (Warning: Pyrophoric substances ignite spontaneously on contact with air.)

Table 4.17 BASES

Ammonium hydroxide

Bicarbonates, such as salts of potassium bicarbonate and sodium bicarbonate

Calcium hydroxide

Carbonates, such as salts of calcium carbonate and sodium carbonate

Potassium hydroxide

Sodium hydroxide

Table 4.18 LIGHT-SENSITIVE CHEMICALS

Bromine

Ethyl ether

Ferric ammonium citrate

Hydrobromic acid

Mercurous nitrate

Mercury salts such as mercuric chloride and mercuric iodide

Oleic acid

Potassium ferrocyanide

Silver salts such as silver acetate and silver chloride

Sodium iodide

Table 4.19 PEROXIDE-FORMING CHEMICALS

Acetaldehyde

Acrylaldehyde

Crotonaldehyde

Cyclohexene

p-Dioxane

Ethyl ether

Isopropyl ether

Potassium peroxide

Tetrahydrofuran

Figure 4.8 SPECIAL INSTRUCTIONS FOR STORING ACIDS

Strong acids should be stored away from alkalis and from each other.

Organic acids such as:
formic acid, glacial acetic acid, acetic acid

must be stored away from

Inorganic acids such as:
nitric acid, sulfuric acid, and hydrochloric acid

Always store acids below counter level to prevent blindness in the event of an accident.

Table 4.20   SOLID AND LIQUID WATER-REACTIVE CHEMICALS

SOLIDS	LIQUIDS
Aluminum chloride (anhydrous)	Acetyl chloride
Calcium carbide	Chlorosulfonic acid
Calcium oxide	Phosphorous trichloride
Ferrous sulfide	Silicon tetrachloride
Lithium*	Stannic chloride
Maleic anhydride	Sulfur chloride
Magnesium	Sulfuryl chloride
Phosphorous pentachloride	Thionyl chloride
Phosphorous pentasulfide	
Potassium*	
Sodium*	

Should be stored under kerosene.

4.5.9 H   CARCINOGENS

- All containers must be labeled as "cancer suspect agents" or "known carcinogen."
- Store according to hazardous properties of the chemical. Table 4.21 lists some of the common carcinogens.
- Use appropriate security when necessary. (See also 4.3.4 G.)

4.5.9 I   TERATOGENS

- All containers must be labeled as "teratogens."
- Store according to hazardous properties of the chemicals. Table 4.21 lists some common teratogens used in laboratories.
- Use appropriate security where necessary.

4.5.9 J   TOXIC COMPOUNDS

These compounds are extremely dangerous to health and life when inhaled, swallowed, or absorbed by skin contact. Use appropriate precautionary measures to avoid exposure. Store according to hazardous properties of the compounds (Table 4.22). Keep emergency medical information phone numbers readily available

4.5.9 K   OXIDIZERS (TABLE 4.15)

- Keep away from reducing agents such as zinc, alkaline metals, and formic acid.
- Keep away from flammable and combustible materials.

Table 4.21   CARCINOGENS AND TERATOGENS COMMONLY STORED IN LABORATORIES

CARCINOGENS	TERATOGENS
Acrylonitrile	Aniline
Antimony compounds	Benzene
Arsenic compounds	Carbon disulfide
Benzene	Carbon monoxide
Benzidine	Chlorinated hydrocarbons
Beryllium	Lead
B-naphthylamine	Mercury
Cadmium compounds	Nitrobenzene
Chloroform	Phosphorus
Chromates, salts of	Radioactive material
Dimethyl sulfate	Toluene
Dioxane	Turpentine
Ethylene dibromide	
Hydrazine	
Nickel carbonyl	
Nickel compounds	
Vinyl chloride	

- Store in dry, cool place. Tables 4.23, 4.24, and 4.25 list incompatible chemicals, commonly used chemical synonyms, and relatively harmless chemicals under normal laboratory storage conditions, respectively.[3,5,9]

4.5.10   CHEMICAL INVENTORY CONTROL

Laboratories must maintain accurate and up-to-date inventories of their chemical supplies. Clearly mandated by the Hazard Communication Standard, chemical inventories provide an excellent mechanism for cost controls as well as efficient use of resources. (Unused chemicals can represent as much as 40% of the hazardous waste generated in laboratories.[7]) Accurate inventories in turn minimize storage space required, security measures necessary, and disposal costs.

Table 4.22   TOXIC COMPOUNDS

SOLIDS	LIQUIDS	GASES
Antimony compounds	Aniline	Carbon monoxide
Arsenic compounds	Bromine	Chlorine
Barium compounds	Carbon disulfide	Cyanogen
Beryllium compounds	Carbon tetrachloride	Diborane
Cadmium compounds	Chloroform	Formaldehyde
Calcium oxide	Chromic acid	Hydrogen bromide
Chromates, salts of	p-Dioxane	Hydrogen chloride
Cyanides, salts of	Ethylene glycol	Hydrogen cyanide
Fluorides, salts of	Formic acid	Hydrogen sulfide
Iodine	Hydrazine	Nitrogen dioxide
Lead compounds	Hydrobromic acid	Ozone
Mercuric compounds	Hydrochloric acid	Sulfur dioxide
Oxalic acid	Hydrofluoric acid	
Pentasulfide	Hydrogen peroxide	
Picric acid	Mercury	
Phenol	Nitric acid	
Phosphorus	Perchloric acid	
Phosphorus, yellow	Phosphorous trichloride	
Phosphorous pentasulfide	Sulfuric acid	
Potassium	Tetrachloroethane	
Selenium compounds	Tetrachlorethylene	
Silver nitrate		
Sodium		
Sodium hydroxide		
Sodium hypochlorite		

Table 4.23   INCOMPATIBLE CHEMICALS*

CHEMICAL	AVOID CONTACT WITH
Acetic acid	Chromic acid, nitric acid, hydroxyl compounds, ethylene glycol, peroxides, perchloric acid, permanganates
Acetic anhydride	Hydroxyl compounds, ethylene glycol, perchloric acid
Acetone	Concentrated nitric and sulfuric acid mixtures
Aluminum, powdered	Water, carbon tetrachloride, other chlorinated hydrocarbons, carbon dioxide, halogens
Ammonia, anhydrous	Mercury, chlorine, iodine, bromine, calcium hypochlorite, hydrofluoric acid (anhydrous)
Ammonium nitrate	Acids, metal powders, flammable liquids, chlorates, nitrates, sulfur, finely divided organic, combustive material
Aniline	Nitric acid, hydrogen peroxide
Bromine	Ammonia, acetylene, butadiene, butane, methane, propane, hydrogen, sodium carbide, turpentine, benzene, finely divided metals
Calcium oxide	Water
Carbon, activated	Calcium hypochlorite, all oxidizing agents
Chlorates	Ammonium salts, acids, metal powder, sulfur, finely divided organic, combustible material
Chromic acid (chromium trioxide)	Acetic acid, naphthalene, camphor, glycerin, turpentine, alcohol, and flammable liquids in general
Chlorine	Same as bromine
Chlorine dioxide	Ammonia, methane, phopine, hydrogen sulfide
Copper	Acetylene, hydrogen peroxide
Cumene hydroperoxide	Acids, organic or inorganic
Flammable liquids	Ammonium nitrate, chromic acid, hydrogen peroxide, nitric acid, sodium peroxide, halogens
Fluorine	Isolate from everything
Hydrazine	Hydrogen peroxide, nitric acid, any other oxidant
Hydrocarbons (butane, propane, benzene, gasoline, turpentine)	Nitric acid, alkali
Hydrofluoric acid, anhydrous	Ammonia, aqueous or anhydrous
Hydrogen peroxide	Copper, chromium, iron, most metals or their salts, alcohol, acetone, organic materials, aniline, nitromethane, flammable or combustible materials
Hydrogen sulfide	Fuming nitrate acid, oxidizing gases
Iodine	Acetylene, ammonia (aqueous or anhydrous), hydrogen
Magnesium, powdered	Water, carbon tetrachloride or other chlorinated hydrocarbons, carbon dioxide, halogens
Mercury	Acetylene, tulminic acid, ammonia
Nitric acid, concentrated	Acetic acid, aniline, chromic acid, hydrocyanic acid, hydrogen sulfide, flammable liquids, flammable gases

Nitroparaffins	Inorganic bases, amines
Oxalic acid	Silver, mercury
Perchloric acid	Acetic anhydride, bismuth and its alloys, alcohol, paper, wood
Peroxides, organic	Acids, avoid friction, store cold
Potassium	Glycerine, ethylene glycol, sulfuric acid, benzaldehyde, carbon tetrachloride, carbon dioxide, water
Potassium chlorate	Sulfuric and other acids
Potassium perchlorate	Sulfuric and other acids
Potassium permanganate	Glycerine, ethylene glycol, sulfuric acid, benzaldehyde
Silver	Acetylene, oxalic acid, tartaric acid, ammonium compounds
Sodium	Carbon tetrachloride, carbon dioxide, water, halogens
Sodium nitrate	Ammonium nitrate and other ammonium salts
Sodium peroxide	Ethyl or methyl alcohol, glacial acetic acid, acetic anhydride, benzaldehyde, carbon disulfide, glycerine, ethyleneglycol, ethyl acetate, methylacetate, turtural
Sulfuric acid	Potassium chlorate, potassium perchlorate, potassium permanganate, or compounds with similar light metals such as sodium or lithium

See also Asiedu S. Incompatible chemicals: an issue to consider. Miles Inc Tech Bull. *1983;13(3):205-207.*

Table 4.24 CHEMICAL SYNONYMS

Acetic acid	Vinegar acid, methanecarboxylic acid, ethanoic acid
Chloroform	Methenyl trichloride, trichloromethane
Chromic acid	Chromic trioxide, chromic anhydride
Ethyl ether	Diethyl oxide, diethyl ether, sulfuric ether, ether
Formaldehyde	Formic aldehyde, methanol, oxymethylene
Hydrogen peroxide	Hydrogen dioxide
Formic acid	Hydrogen carboxylic acid, methanoic acid
Nitric acid	Aqua fortis, azotic acid, engravers acid
Picric acid	Nitrooxantic acid, phenoitrinitrate, picronitric acid, trinitrophenol
Sulfuric acid	Battery acid, hydrogen sulfate toluene, methylbenzene, phenylmethane
Xylene	Dimethylbenzene

Table 4.25 RELATIVELY HARMLESS CHEMICALS UNDER NORMAL LABORATORY STORAGE
CONDITIONS

Aluminum sheets	Aluminum potassium sulfate (alum)	Aluminum sulfate
Ammonium chloride	Ammonium molybdate	Ammonium sulfate
Bismuth nitrate	Butyric acid	Cadmium
Calcium acetate	Calcium acid phosphate (diabasic)	Calcium carbonate (marble chips)
Calcium chloride	Calcium oxide	Calcium sulfate
Charcoal, activated	Charcoal, animal	Charcoal, wood
Citric acid	Cobalt chloride	Collodion
Copper metal	Copper, sheet, soft	Copper, wire
Cotton, absorbent	Cupric oxide	Dextrin, white powder
Ethyl acetate	Ferric ammonium citrate	Ferric chloride
Ferrous sulfate	Gelatin, granular	Graphite
Iron metal filings	Iron sulfide	Koalin
Lead sheet	Lead oxide (mono)	Litmus
Lycopodium	Magnesium oxide	Magnesium dioxide
Methyl orange indicator	Oil, cottonseed	Paraffin
Phenolphthalein	Potassium bitartrate	Potassium bromide
Potassium chloride	Potassium sulfate	Pumice
Resorcinol	Salicylic acid	Soap, castile
Sodium acetate, fused	Sodium alum	Sodium bicarbonate
Sodium bisulfate	Sodium bisulfite	Sodium borate
Sodium carbonate	Sodium chloride	Sodium phosphate
Sodium potassium tartrate	Sodium sulfate	Sodium thiosulfate
Starch	Steel wool	Sugar, dextrose
Sugar, sucrose	Tartaric acid	Zinc metal, mossy
Zinc strips	Zinc sulfate	

4.5.10 A BENEFITS OF CHEMICAL INVENTORY MANAGEMENT
- Controlled chemical inventories provide more opportunities for chemical exchange between laboratory departments or sections.
- Minimization of purchases provides smaller containers that are less hazardous to personnel. Smaller containers break less frequently than do larger ones, and spillage and cleanup is less hazardous.
- Smaller purchases result in use of fresh chemicals, unopened containers, with original labels intact.
- Excess chemical storage results in increased demands of maintenance expense and personnel.
- Chemical tracking and inventory control facilitates federally mandated hazardous waste control and management by reducing chemical amounts to be collected, separated, packaged, labeled, and recorded for waste disposal (Figure 4.9).

4.5.10 B EFFECTIVE INVENTORY CONTROL
- Proper disposal of any chemical that is no longer used
- Proper disposal of any chemical that is out of date
- On-going program to reduce quantities maintained in stock
- Chemical tracking to prevent duplication of purchases
- Comprehensive file or data system for maintenance of records. Data systems utilizing bar code labeling are increasingly successful; computer-based inventory systems are widely used.
- Records of chemicals with their ultimate disposal requirements
- Regularly scheduled inspections of storage facilities for potential hazards such as leaks or inappropriate storage conditions
- Cooperation of all personnel in maintaining an accurate inventory

4.6 HAZARDS IN THE LABORATORY

4.6.1 CHEMICAL SPILLS

4.6.1 A CHEMICAL SPILL CLEANUP PROCEDURES[5]
Remember, a 1-gallon spill equals 20 square feet! The following list includes the cleanup procedures to be followed in the event of an accidental spill of a hazardous chemical in the laboratory.
- Notify immediate supervisor about the spill.
- Evacuate all nonessential personnel from the spill area.
- Determine, if possible, the chemical spilled and estimate the quantity.
- If the spilled material is flammable, turn off ignition, heat sources, and ventilation systems.
- Contain the spill using a bag of absorbent on the spill site, as appropriate. Individual chemical containment may vary with the severity of the hazard. Consider specific chemical hazard instructions.
- Immediately notify the chemical hygiene officer and the laboratory director so that the spill response team may be activated, if appropriate.

Figure 4.9 CHEMICAL INVENTORY FORM

Laboratory _____ Location _____

Department _____ Verified by _____

Chemical Name (Not formula)	Location				Amount Stored Monthly	Hazard Class				
	CC	RE	FL	Other		H	F	R	C	Other

CC = chemical storage cabinet   RE= refrigerator   FL= flammable cabinet

(H) Health

0. Ordinary combustible

1. Slightly hazardous

2. Hazardous

3. Extreme danger

4. Deadly

(F) Fire hazard

0. Will not harm

1. Ignites if preheated

2. Ignites if moderately heated

3. Ignites at most ambient conditions

(R) Reactivity

0. Stable and not reactive

1. Unstable if heated

2. Violent change

3. Shock and heat may detonate

4. May detonate

(C) Corrosivity

OXY - oxidizer

ACID - acid

ALK - alkali

COR - corrosive

W - use no water

RAD - radioactive

- Individuals working directly with the spill shall wear all appropriate PPE; respirator or SCBA, protective gloving; long-sleeved, moisture-resistant gown; coverall; chemical splash goggles if SCBA is not used; and protective boots or shoe covers.
- Clean up the spill if appropriate. This procedure should be carried out by the designated safety officer or trained personnel in that area.[10]

4.6.1 B   SPILL TEAM RESPONSE[5]

- Attend to any persons who have been contaminated or injured.
- Persons with caustics on their skin or eyes should be immediately assisted in utilizing emergency shower/eye wash (a period of 15 minutes). Contaminated clothing must be removed immediately.
- Any employee coming in contact with any chemical will be assisted to the emergency department or medical professional for evaluation and/or treatment.
- Confine or contain the spill to a small area. Do not let it spread.
- Utilize designated spill kits including spill containment materials such as vermiculite, dry sand, or spill pillow. For inorganic acids or bases, use neutralizing agents or an absorbent mixture such as soda ash or diatomaceous earth.
- Carefully remove and clean any cartons or bottles that have been dropped. Do not attempt to pick up or move broken glass or other sharps, rather, use a broom and dust pan for handling such articles.
- Sweep up moisture-absorbent material or remove spill pillows and properly dispose of them in a clearly marked leak-proof bag or other disposable container. Caustics will be neutralized before disposal. Additional precautions such as use of a vacuum cleaner equipped with a HEPA-filter may be necessary to clean up spills of more highly toxic solids. Broken glass or sharps should first be placed in a rigid plastic or cardboard container before being disposed of.
- Dispose of residues in a similar safe fashion and adequately ventilate the area before allowing personnel to return to the work area.
- Clean up safety equipment and return it to its designated storage place. Replace any disposable components, such as absorbents, spills kits.
- Fill out and complete appropriate documentation of the incident/accident. Evaluate and follow up as a preventive measure against future incidents.

4.6.1 C   DECONTAMINATION OF POTENTIALLY INFECTIOUS SPILLS[10]

- Clear area of all nonessential personnel, advise supervisor of situation.
- Wear PPE—gloves, gown, apron, face shield, shoe covers.
- Absorb bulk of spilled material, pick up broken glass or fragments using tongs or broom-dust pan technique.
- Clean spill site with detergent; household detergent will do.
- Disinfect spill site thoroughly (1:10 bleach solution).
- Rinse well with water and dry spill site.
- Dispose of all contaminated materials as biohazardous waste.

4.6.1 D   TRAINING PERSONNEL IN SPILL PROCEDURES

The OSHA requirements under 29 CFR 1910.120 (q)—Hazardous Waste Operations and Emergency Response (HAZWOPER)—have placed a responsibility on laboratories to address certain aspects of the law. Worker safety is the responsibility of OSHA mandates while control of hazardous waste is not. However, when the workers' safety may be compromised, it is appropriate that procedures reflect the HAZWOPER standard requirements. The regulation requires training of employees who are designated as spill responders at one or more of five levels. These training requirements include:

- *Level One—First Responder (Awareness Level)*: Personnel who do not perform cleanup activities, but might be a "first responder" on the scene of a spill. This level may represent any level of laboratory worker and it addresses hazardous materials awareness—being able to identify materials that are involved and inform appropriate personnel.
- *Level Two —First Responder (Operations Level)*: This level represents those workers who respond defensively to a release of material by stopping the source such as shutting off a leaking formalin container. This level also stresses hazardous materials awareness and may also represent a number of laboratory positions.
- *Level Three —Hazardous Materials Technician*: This level represents those workers who actually participate in spill cleanup. Training requirements include familiarity with chemical hazards, PPE, and cleanup techniques. This level of action requires a minimum of 24 hours of training under the HAZWOPER standard.
- *Level Four—Hazardous Materials Technician*: This is essentially the same as level three, with additional technical abilities needed and local and regional reporting also being necessary.
- *Level Five—On-Scene Incident Commander*: This level represents senior managers who would coordinate activities in the event of a major incident. A minimum of 24 hours' training is required with knowledge of local and regional emergency planning and response agencies.

The major portion of this law does not apply to the average medical laboratory. Laboratory personnel who routinely work with chemical hazards such as xylene, formaldehyde, and a number of other hazardous materials should be competent to handle an emergency situation involving those materials. Proper employee training for these situations is mandated by the Laboratory Standard.[11] Unless the spill represents an unusual situation, most laboratory spills will represent a minor "controlled" spill and the laboratory personnel should be competent to handle the cleanup procedure. This regulation may be applicable to those facilities that have designated "spill teams" to respond to certain hazardous chemical spills. It is up to employers to become knowledgeable about HAZWOPER requirements for training so that they can determine an appropriate program for spill control. However, one way or another, it is prudent to consider certain factors regarding spill procedures:

- A potentially harmful incident should be handled by properly trained personnel.
- Facilities should anticipate how they will handle a variety of incident conditions.
- Facilities can determine whether or not they want to work with outside contractors to control spills or handle problems in-house.
- Protection of employees as well as the potential liability involved in the event of injury to cleanup personnel who have not been adequately trained should be carefully considered.

4.6.2   FLAMMABLE LIQUID HAZARDS IN THE LABORATORY[12]

A review of NFPA statistics demonstrates that very frequently fires in laboratories are the result of ignition of vapor from a flammable liquid. This fact emphasizes the need for regular evaluation of procedures for handling, use, and storage of flammables because of their greater potential for creating fire hazards in the workplace. An evaluation of these potential hazards, a plan for storage of the materials, determination of appropriate disposal techniques, and establishment of a comprehensive spill or leak control plan will substantially reduce the hazard of flammable liquids in the laboratory.

4.6.2 A   PERFORM A SAFETY SURVEY OF LABORATORY HAZARDS

- Eliminate procedures or faulty equipment that might permit a release of vapors.
- Establish a checklist to record information of safety procedures required and the location of safety equipment.
- Decide whether it is necessary to conduct a global survey (the entire laboratory) or surveys directed functionally by usage (storage, transfer, use, and disposal) of hazardous materials.
- Each laboratory section should be considered a separate unit and surveyed accordingly.
- These guidelines for surveys also provide information regarding the most economical use of both materials and equipment. More effective methods of storage and use of flammable materials often results in significant savings in the costs of labor, materials, disposal, and safety equipment.

4.6.2 B   STORAGE OF FLAMMABLE LIQUIDS

Decentralize storage of hazardous liquids. NFPA code 45 requires that storage cabinets must be used if more than 10 gallons of class I and II liquids are stored in 100 feet of floor area. There must be no more than three safety cabinets in the same 100-foot area with other flammable liquids. Storage cabinets must be of double-wall construction, with 1.5 inches of insulating air space in walls, door, top, and floor, and three-point locking doors. Vent openings must have caps in place or the lower vent must be connected to an approved exhaust system. Flame arrester screens in vent openings must be intact. A 2-inch spill-leak sill must be in place.

Safety cabinets for storing acids and corrosive material must:
- Be made of metal or wood construction.
- Have a chemical-resistant coating.
- Have polyethylene shelf liners.

"Piggyback" metal cabinets for either acids or flammables:
- Can be mounted on top of standard 30-gallon metal cabinets. (Acids, however, should never be stored above counter level.)
- Permit segregated storage of corrosive chemicals at same location as flammable liquids without requiring additional floor space.

Safety cans must:
- Be leak-tight and should automatically relieve pressure at 5 psig.
- Have flame arrester for spout.
- Close automatically after use.
- Be checked for impairment regularly (leakage, pressure release, self-closure).

• Have springs or self-closure that must not be tampered with.

Figure 4.10 lists some of the mandated requirements for the storage of flammable liquids. Laboratories should, however, consult more detailed text for specific chemical classifications, flash points, and other pertinent information.[11]

4.6.2 C   DISPOSAL PROCEDURES
• Most common source of unsafe conditions. If waste is enough to warrant a waste-solvent drum, it must be in a storage cabinet connected to a solid earth ground and bonded to each container that is emptied. The drum should have an approved fill vent/funnel installed for safe pours.
• Safety disposal cans should be inspected as laboratory safety cans. Use plastic disposal cans because they are more damage resistant.
• No solvent wastes are to be disposed of in a sewer system.
• Solvent-soaked towels, rags, or absorbent materials should be stored in approved air-tight waste cans, and emptied on a regular basis.

4.6.2 D   SPILL CONTROL
Equipment for spill control:
• Must be adequate for volume of flammable liquid in the area.
• Includes spill squeegees and spill absorbents.
• Includes spill waste disposal compliance with local fire codes. Check waste hauler services for bonding and qualifications.

Personnel must be trained for spill control.

Suitable PPE, including respirators, eye, hand, foot, and body protection must be included.

Figure 4.10   STORAGE REQUIREMENTS FOR FLAMMABLE LIQUIDS [21]

The NFPA Code 45 sets limits for flammable liquid containers outside storage cabinets. Most flammble medical laboratory reagents are limited to no more than a total of 10 gallons of flammable liquid stored outside safety cabinets. This amount also corresponds to the College of American Pathologists Guidelines.

OSHA Section 1910.106-d-3 General Industrial Standard specifies the amount of chemical containers that may be stored inside a storage cabinet. No more than a total of 60 gallons of flammable liquid can be stored in a single flammable storage cabinet.

Maximum container sizes:	Class 1A	1B	1C
Glass or approved plastic	1 Pint	1 Quart	1 Gallon
Metals cans	1 Gallon	5 Gallons	5 Gallons

4.6.3 EXPLOSIONS IN THE LABORATORY[1]

A number of chemicals capable of creating an explosion are commonly used in the laboratory. Identification of these hazards is essential, and appropriate guidelines for use, handling, and disposal are vital.

- *Benzene*: May explode in combination with oxidants.
- *Ether*: Forms explosive peroxides on exposure to air and light.
- *Chromic Acid*: Explosive with acetic acid, acetic anhydride; may ignite with acetone, glycerol, methanol, butanol, ethanol, and pyridine.
- *Glycerol*: Violent or explosive reactions with oxidizing agents.
- *Hydrogen Peroxide*: Highly dangerous because when heated, shocked, or contaminated, the concentrated material can explode or start fires.
- *Methanol*: A solvent that is both highly flammable and explosive on impact.
- *Nitrocellulose*: Highly explosive when dry, highly flammable (celloidin, collodion, embedding media).
- *Perchloric Acid*: Like acids, can burn and corrode. Potentially explosive above 70% concentration; reacts violently with acetic acid, alcohols, formaldehyde, dehydrative agents, carbon, ether, glycols, and iodides.
- *Picric Acid*: Stronger explosive than TNT. Must be kept out of contact with metals. Readily detonates when dry, explosive in greater than 50% solutions with water, forms heat, friction, or impact-sensitive salts with many metals (lead, mercury, copper, zinc). Never use picric acid near an open flame. (See 4.3.5 A, 4.3.5 E, and 4.6.5.)
- *Potassium Dichromate*: Reacts violently with hydroxylamine.
- *Potassium Permanganate*: Explosive when combined with acetic acid, acetic anhydride, hydrochloric acid, or sulfuric acids; causes fires when combined with glycerol and solid potassium permanganate.
- *Silver Nitrate*: May explode when combined with ethanol or charcoal.

This is only a partial list of the many chemical substances that can cause explosions in the laboratory. There are numerous chemicals that, when heated, shocked, or contaminated, can create extremely hazardous reactions. Always consult the chemical MSDS for complete information before using or handling any chemical or beginning any new procedure.

4.6.4 HEALTH HAZARDS IN THE ELECTRON MICROSCOPY AND PLASTICS LABORATORY[13]

As a unit of any institution, the electron microscopy laboratory contains some of the most hazardous chemical substances to be found in any laboratory. Because of the frequent interaction between laboratories, particularly in matters of fixation, it is appropriate that chemical hazards frequently existing in electron microscopy procedures be identified and personnel receive appropriate training in these hazards. Table 4.26 lists some of the common hazards of the electron microscopy and plastics laboratory.

4.6.4 A EMBEDDING MEDIA
The primary health hazard–related concerns are those substances that may be carcinogenic or potential carcinogens, primary irritants, or those that may produce allergic responses, and toxic substances. Each product should be very carefully

examined for potential hazardous characteristics. Examples of popular embedding media (Ted Pella Inc) include the following:

Epoxy (routine use): Eponate 12, Medcast, Araldites, Maraglass 655
Epoxy (low viscosity): Spurr, Quetols, Pelco Ultra-low Viscosity
Epoxy (water miscible): Quetols
Melamine (water miscible): Nanoplast
Polar Acrylic: LR White, LR Gold, Lowicryls, butyl methacrylate, methyl methacrylate
Acrylic (methacrylates, water miscible): Pelco GMA, PEG-GMA kit

4.6.4 B   GUIDELINES FOR SAFE USE

All materials used in electron and light microscopy laboratories should be handled with great care. Precautions should be used for acrylic polyester as well as epoxy media.[14] Suggestions for precautions include the following:

- MSDSs on all reagents and media must be readily available and understood.
- The area used for plastic techniques should be restricted.
- Vigilant use of an efficient fume hood is an absolute requirement. It is important that all preparation of the medium be performed under a hood.
- Safety goggles, with side shields, must always be worn when preparing media.
- Contact lenses should not be worn in the plastic techniques laboratory. Plastics have been known to react with certain lens types.

Table 4.26   HAZARDS IN ELECTRON MICROSCOPY AND PLASTICS LABORATORIES

MEDIA	HAZARD
FIXATIVES	
Glutaraldehyde	Toxic, corrosive, irritant, corneal damage
Osmium tetroxide	Extremely toxic, vapors, fumes, hazardous waste
Buffers	
Cacodylic acid	Extremely toxic, contains arsenic
DYES/STAINS	
Uranyl acetate	Radioactive
Lead	Highly toxic
Dehydrating/Infiltrating Solvents	Irritants, absorbed through skin, flammable
Methanol	Flammable, poison
Ethanol	Flammable, poison
Acetone	Flammable, poison
Propylene oxide	Corneal burns, may be a carcinogen
Dimethylformamide	Toxic to the liver
Styrene	Damages central nervous system
2,2, Dimethoxypropane (DMP)	Extremely flammable

- Disposable jackets, aprons, or laboratory coats are to be used.
- Plastic media permeate rubber or latex gloves. Most gloves offer little or no real protection because the permeation rates of the media vary greatly from glove type to glove type. A double-glove technique may be used. Some technologists use both protective barrier creams for their hands and gloves, while others use barrier creams, a light cotton glove, and a rubber or latex glove. It is difficult to determine which method offers more protection. It is important for technologists to avoid any direct contact with the media, especially in the liquid form and fumes.
- When removing gloves, first pull the finger tips loose, then shake the gloves directly into an appropriate waste container.
- Frequent hand washing with soap and cold water is suggested as a further precaution. DO NOT use an organic solvent such as alcohol to clean your hands or work surfaces. The solvent breaks down the protective lipid barrier of the skin.
- Unpolymerized material, sometimes found around freshly embedded blocks, is especially toxic and contact must be avoided.
- Brown paper spread over the immediate work surface readily indicates any spills that may occur and will help prevent accidental direct contact with any unpolymerized splatters or droplets.
- Use disposable materials and supplies, never glass or washables for processing specimens. Disposable containers reduce contamination.
- Use forceps or tongs to handle newly formed blocks. This technique minimizes direct contact with the media.
- All containers should remain covered when not directly in use.
- If possible, the embedding oven should be vented to the hood.
- Tops should be placed on BEEM and gelatin capsules. Molds should be placed in closed Petri dishes.
- All transfers of components, infiltration, and embedding mixtures between containers should be done using disposable pipettes.
- If possible, avoid spilling any of the chemical. If contamination should occur, rinse hands or the area well with water, followed by a thorough soap and water wash. Do not use alcohol.
- Dispose of all utensils and other waste materials in double-lined waste bags, tied securely, and labeled clearly for disposal according to the facility guidelines.
- If any unusual rash, burning sensation, or respiratory discomfort is noted, consult a physician immediately.

Disposal of unpolymerized embedding waste includes the following:
- Infiltrating and embedding mixture wastes should be considered hazardous.
- All contaminated utensils should be considered hazardous.
- Media such as epoxy, acrylic, and polyester must be kept separate because of potentially explosive chemical incompatibilities.
- Flammable hazards occur with infiltrating mixtures of resin and alcohol, acetone, or propylene oxide and should be dealt with accordingly.

Environmental Concerns: The laboratory should direct particular concern to the substances that may cause in-house contamination or pollution as well as those that may represent a distinct fire hazard. It is essential that proper handling and disposal procedures for these substances be carefully followed.

4.6.4 C ALLERGIC RESPONSES TO CHEMICAL USE

Many technologists working with materials frequently used in the electron microscopy or plastics laboratory have demonstrated allergic reactions or hypersensitivity responses to these materials.[15] More recently, allergic reactions to wearing latex gloves have initiated a medical alert by the Food and Drug Administration to inform health care workers of the potential hazards of latex glove use (see also Chapter 9).[16] The reactions to the use of plastic embedding media and latex gloves are very similar. These reactions have been demonstrated primarily on the fingers and hands but more serious responses, including respiratory distress, have also been documented.[15] Allergic responses may be caused by the formation of antibodies when inhalation or skin penetration occurs with exposure to infiltrating or embedding mixtures. These responses may cause airway, skin, or systemic hypersensitization of exposed personnel. These infiltrating or embedding mixtures become more volatile due to diluent action and the solvent component of the mixture breaks down the lipid barriers of the skin, making penetration of the mixtures more rapid. Reactions may range from localized dermatitis to fatal anaphylactic responses. Methods for the prevention of exposure to these allergens and minimization of allergic responses must be instituted into laboratory health and safety programs.

4.6.5 PICRIC ACID[17]

Picric acid (2,4,6-trinitrophenol) is a highly sensitive chemical that, when dry, may explode if exposed to friction, shock, or sudden heating. It has an explosive nature more powerful than TNT. Because of the extremely hazardous nature of this chemical, certain characteristics regarding use and handling of picric acid must be clearly understood.

Picric acid forms salts on contact with metals and heavy metal picrates that are also highly sensitive to detonation. It must not be mixed with zinc or mercury salts. Early reports of detonation may have been the result of minute quantities of a metal picrate in the threads of a metal-capped container. Picric acid is now sold only in plastic-capped containers to prevent this from happening. However, even with a plastic cap, the acid may dry out over a period of time and become highly dangerous.

If drying occurs in a plastic-capped container, follow these steps:
*   Immerse the bottle upside down in water for a few hours to wet the threads of the container.
*   The bottle can then be opened and filled with water.
*   Allow the water-filled bottle to stand 2 to 4 days to ensure complete wetting of the acid contents.
*   At this point, the container and contents can be disposed of by a commercial disposal service.
*   Metal-capped containers should be handled by a trained expert, such as a bomb squad member.[3]

Picric acid is not only a serious potential explosive chemical but is also absorbed through the skin and is toxic. Individuals handling this chemical should wear chemically resistant gloves such as neoprene or nitrile. The best advice is to eliminate the use of picric acid altogether if possible.[7]

One of the problems associated with procedures using picric acid may be the origin and date of publication of the procedure. For instance, technologists are very familiar with the use of some chemicals and procedures that have been demonstrated to be long-term health hazards, such as xylene. Further, procedures that may have been appropriate in the past, such as handling specimens without gloves, have been found to be a health or safety hazard. For example, in the well-respected book, *The Theory and Practice of Histotechnology,* Sheehan and Hrapchak (1980) describe the procedure of dehydrating picric acid for use in a Gram stain.[18(p234)] This procedure is no longer recommended. Although a note was included in the text that anhydrous picric acid has explosive tendencies, this risk is not acceptable in light of alternative methods.

The use of picric acid can be moderated by:
• Purchasing only the amounts necessary and making sure it is maintained in a moist environment.
• Purchasing commercially prepared solutions to fit your needs, eliminating the use of crystal picric acid altogether.

It must be understood that the use of picric acid in the laboratory is not a violation of any regulation. What is mandated is the proper use, handling, and disposal of any hazardous chemical in the laboratory. If these standards are maintained, there should be no concern when an inspection is made of your facilities.

4.6.6 MERCURY

Most of our laboratories have now clearly come to understand the major health hazards presented by the use of mercury. From earliest times, events linking mercuric poisoning have occurred with tragic consequences—the death of Sir Isaac Newton at age 50 years was probably due to mercury poisoning; early hat makers, using mercuric nitrite solutions to cure felt were commonly described as "mad as hatters." Remember the Mad Hatter in *Alice in Wonderland*? Patients treated for syphilis in the 16th century were subjected to mercury massages and more recently, the tragic poisoning of entire fishing villages in Japan are reported to have resulted from industrial dumping of methyl mercury waste into Minamata Bay.[19]

The ombudsman office of the EPA states that there is no ban on the disposal of mercury via landfills in the USA (Spring 1994). Furthermore, there are landfills in the USA that are permitted to accept any form of waste mercury. Generators should contact their state or regional EPA office for the names of approved facilities (J Dapson, personal communication). However, there is a catch to landfill disposal—it is very expensive. To rid your laboratory of mercury, be prepared to pay the cost. Samples of waste must be submitted to the licensed disposal company for analysis of the mercury concentration. The level of mercury present determines the appropriate treatment and also the cost of disposal (see regulations). Any way you look at it, disposal of mercury is a very expensive proposition (if you can find a disposal service that will even take it). Although many landfills are licensed to accept mercury, they will not because it is not cost-effective for them to do so. There is no law mandating that landfills must accept everything for which they are licensed. Beware of unscrupulous waste disposal services and landfills. Ultimately, the generator (laboratory) can be liable. One facility that used a small landfill to dispose of "nonhazardous" waste was held responsible for waste that was contaminated by improperly stored hazardous waste, caused by the disposal service, that leached mercury into the nonhazardous waste area. Still other problems have been described where laboratories known to have mercury contamination have had to go through exhaustive procedures to rid their facilities of mercury sources such as cleaning all the elbows and joints in the plumbing lines and replacing metal baskets and sink rims.[20]

4.6.6 A   REGULATIONS
- Must be handled as a hazardous waste.
- Must be sent to the facility for reclamation in retort or roasting thermal process unit.
- *Recovery methods*: Commercially very expensive; there are no methods of recovery for laboratory use other than precipitation (see 4.6.6 E) to reduce volume of waste.
- Most mercury waste lies in laboratory storage for indefinite periods because of expensive or inaccessible disposal services.

4.6.6 B   SOURCES OF MERCURY WASTE
- Surplus reagents and waste reagents containing mercury
- Old equipment containing mercury compounds
- Manometer and thermometers

4.6.6 C   WASTE MINIMIZATION
- Encourage use of alternatives for reagents such as zinc formalin fixatives.
- Wherever mercury is used, encourage facility redistribution programs.
- Collect liquid mercury in metal shipping flasks and send to commercial facility.
- *Thermometers and manometers*[21]: Use alternative instruments such as red alcohol or mineral spirit-filled thermometers.
  - Use Teflon-coated, where mercury thermometers are essential.
  - Replace thermometers with thermocouples in physics laboratories.
  - Replace manometers with pressure transducers in engineering experiments.
  - Use bimetal or stainless steel thermometers in heating and cooling units.
  - Try stainless steel or digital thermometers in other laboratory situations.
- *Mercury reagents*: Replace mercury-contaminated fixatives such as Harris hematoxylin stain with a non–mercury-containing hematoxylin stain formula, and Zenkers's, Helly's, Ohlmacher's, Carnoy-Lebrun, B-5, or Shardin's fixatives with mercuric chloride–free fixatives such as zinc formalin fixatives.
  - When used as a biocide, mercuric chloride can be replaced with 5% to 10% methylene chloride, 1% formalin, 1 N hydrochloric acid, sodium azide, and sodium hypochlorite.
  - If mercuric chloride is used as a catalyst for reactions, eliminate and let the reaction time run longer.

4.6.6 D   SPILL AND LEAK CONTROL
- Store mercury containers closed, in secondary containers, in well-ventilated area.
- Place instruments or apparatus containing mercury in secondary tray or pan large enough to contain any chemical spill, during moving process.
- Always use a hood when transferring mercury from one container to another. Always use a secondary tray to collect any spillage.
- Any mercury-containing equipment, reagent, or instrument should be provided with spill control and containment devices such as trays.

4.6.6 E PRECIPITATION OF MERCURY WASTE

- Add sodium carbonate to solution to raise the pH to 8.0 or higher.
- Filter the solution, collecting precipitated mercury in the filter paper for the disposal service. The filter paper containing the mercury precipitate can be temporarily stored in secure closed containers until shipment.
- If solution to be treated is with a Zenker's fixative, potassium dichromate must also be disposed of properly. To treat the potassium dichromate:
  - Add sulfuric acid to the dichromate solution to a pH of 1.0.
  - Add solid sodium thiosulfate until the solution becomes cloudy and blue.
  - Let stand overnight, then filter to collect the precipitate for disposal.
  - Dispose of liquid portion of the solution down the drain if other ingredients permit. (Chromium compounds, however, must not be put down any drain!)

4.6.7 DRAIN DISPOSAL OF LABORATORY REAGENTS[22]

Never pour anything down a laboratory drain unless this work practice has been approved by the facility and is in compliance with federal, state, and local agency regulations. Chloroform, chromium, mercury, nickel, phenol, silver, toluene, trichloroethane, and zinc must especially not be poured down drains. The laboratory must consult with the local Publicly Owned Treatment Works (POTWs) (wastewater treatment facilities) before establishing waste disposal procedures. Regulatory agency mandates that affect the laboratory waste disposal operations include the following:

4.6.7 A THE CLEAN WATER ACT (1972)

- Set standards for what the POTWs could accept for treatment.
- Established the National Pretreatment Program (1976), which lists 126 chemicals as toxic pollutants and requires industry to pretreat these wastes prior to discharge into the sewer system.

Although laboratories are not regulated by these standards, it is important to know that the chemicals discharged by laboratories are of concern to the POTWs regardless of their origin.

4.6.7 B GENERAL PRETREATMENT

General pretreatment and national pollutant discharge elimination system regulations (CFR Vol. 55, No. 42, July 24, 1990. 40 CFR Parts 122 and 403) represent a revision of the National Pretreatment Program. The EPA and individual states oversee pretreatment programs of POTWs. The law has a larger impact on small users such as laboratories.

4.6.7 C CHEMICAL DISCHARGES

Chemical discharges prohibited from disposal in a sanitary sewer system include:

- Reagents that pass through the POTW untreated, such as solvents (clearing agents) that are not soluble in water and, therefore unable to be emulsified in the treatment process
- Reagents that interfere with POTW operation such as large amounts of formaldehyde, which disrupt or diminish the activity of the bacterial population necessary for treatment

- Reagents that pose a fire or explosion hazard such as xylene, xylene substitutes, and alcohols
- Reagents that are corrosive (discharges with a pH value less than 5.0), which include decalcifying agents (unless POTW is capable of handling such solutions)
- Discharge that results in gases, vapors, or fumes in quantities that could compromise personnel health such as formaldehyde discharged close to a treatment plant
- Discharge of petroleum oil, cutting oil, or mineral oil products that interfere with the treatment process such as some limonene xylene substitutes that contain mineral oil
- Others, not usually associated with laboratory operation

4.6.7 D NOTIFICATION AND DETERMINATION OF HAZARDOUS WASTE CATEGORY[22]
Most nonresidential users of POTWs must submit at least a one-time notification to the EPA Regional Waste Management Director, the state Hazardous Waste Authority and the local POTW declaring each discharge into the sewer system. This notification must include
- Name of hazardous waste
- EPA hazardous waste number
- Type of discharge (batched for discharge or continuous in flow)

The laboratory must certify that it has a waste management program in place to reduce the volume and toxicity of wastes generated by the laboratory. Discharges less than 15 kg (about 3.5 gallons) of nonacute hazardous waste per month do not have to be reported. Discharges of any quantity of acutely hazardous waste require reporting. There are no histology chemicals which fall in this category.[17] Use of detoxification products for treatment of formaldehyde requires the approval of the local POTW.

The laboratory must determine which reporting category is applicable to its operation. Depending on the size of the laboratory operation and complexity of waste generated, the laboratory should consult with the local authorities for information and assistance. When talking with local authorities, the laboratory should have available information regarding the hazardous waste to be discharged from the facility. The chart in Figure 4.11 should assist in defining a laboratory's reagent and chemical hazardous waste inventory. To calculate chemical waste concentrations, a 1% solution equals 10,000 ppm and 1 g/L equals 1,000 ppm. Remember, when talking with the local POTW, if disposal is denied for a chemical waste and it can be made nonhazardous by laboratory pretreatment, say so. They may give their approval on this basis.[22] Many of these chemicals can be treated, such as decoloration of stains, dilution of alcohols, and removal of heavy metals from solutions.

4.6.7 E DISPOSAL OF DIAMINOBENIZIDINE (DAB) TETRAHYDROCHLORIDE AND MERCURIC CHLORIDE[7]
Appropriate disposal of particularly hazardous chemicals in the laboratory has become increasingly important. Techniques continue to be developed for the safe

handling and removal of these chemicals. Of particular interest to the technologist is the safe disposal of DAB tetrahydrochloride and mercuric chloride.

DAB: DAB tetrahydrochloride is commonly used in immunohistochemistry procedures and is a suspected carcinogen in humans. It has been reported that it creates tumors of the respiratory tract of mice (NIOSH). Early procedures for treating this very dangerous chemical included treating the DAB with bleach. However, this method is not recommended because the resulting chemical product is unknown at the present time. Crookham and Dapson in their book, *Hazardous Chemicals in Histopathology Laboratories,* recommend the following procedure[7]:

- Prepare an aqueous stock solution of 0.2 M potassium permanganate (31.6 g/L) and 2.0 M sulfuric acid (112 mL concentrated acid per liter).
- Dilute the DAB solution to not exceed 0.9 mg/mL.
- For each 10 mL of DAB solution add 5 mL of 0.2 M potassium permanganate and 5 mL of 2.0 M sulfuric acid.
- Allow to stand at least 10 minutes (it is now nonmutagenic).
- Decolorize the mixture with ascorbic acid (add powder until color disappears).
- Neutralize mixture with sodium bicarbonate (test with pH meter or pH paper).
- Discard the solution down the drain if approved by local wastewater authorities.

Figure 4.11   REAGENT AND HAZARDOUS WASTE INVENTORY

Laboratory Section _____   Verified by _____   Date _____

Chemical	Constituents	Hazard	Pretreatment	Untreated	Batch	Flow	Amount/Week	Amount/Month

Mercuric Chloride:
- Precipitate mercury from a mercuric chloride solution. (Never dispose down drain.)
- Add sodium carbonate to solution to raise the pH to 8.0 or higher.
- Filter solution, collecting precipitated mercury for the disposal service.
- If solution to be treated is from Zenker's solution, potassium dichromate must also be disposed of properly. (Chromium compounds must not be put down any drain.) To treat the potassium dichromate:
  - Add sulfuric acid to dichromate solution to pH 1.0.
  - Add solid sodium thiosulfate until solution becomes cloudy and blue.
  - Neutralize with sodium carbonate.
  - Let stand overnight, then filter to collect precipitate for proper disposal.
  - Dispose of liquid down drain if other ingredients permit.

4.6.8   CHEMICAL INJURY OF THE EYE[23]

The single most important treatment for chemical injury to the eye is immediate irrigation of the eye with large amounts of liquid, preferably a pH-correct liquid.

4.6.8 A   ALKALI
Ammonia: Frequently found in bleach and other cleaning solutions, ammonia forms ammonium hydroxide, which penetrates the eye more rapidly than any other alkali. Severe damage may result.
Sodium Hydroxide: Rapidly penetrates the eye, severe damage
Calcium Hydroxide: Less severe injuries
Potassium Hydroxide: Severe damage like sodium hydroxide
Magnesium Hydroxide: Severe damage

4.6.8 B   ACID
Weak or diluted acids cause less damage than alkalis.
Mineral Acids (Sulfuric, Hydrochloric): Severe damage
Heavy Metals (Chromic Acids): Severe damage
Sulfur Dioxide (in bleach and refrigerants) forms sulfurous acid and can cause severe eye damage because of its high lipid and water solubility. It denatures protein and activates numerous enzymes.
Hydrofluoric Acid (Dissolves Cellular Membranes), Chromic Acid, Hydrochloric Acid, and Nitric Acid: Damage results from prolonged exposure to fumes.
Acetic Acid: Severe damage results from prolonged exposure to high concentrations. Concentrations of less than 10% produce much minor damage

4.6.8 C   TOXIC EFFECTS
Depends on anion and cation concentrations. Alkali damage is based on pH caused by hydroxyl ion. Causes swelling and cleavage of collagen fibrils within the cornea. Irreversible damage at a pH higher than 11.5. Corneal ulceration and possible loss of the eye.

4.6.8 D   EMERGENCY TREATMENT
- Copious irrigation of the external eye following a chemical injury is essential.
- Cold tap water is often the only available irrigation solution but may be

extremely discomforting to the victim. A commercially available, pH-balanced physiologic solution is preferred.
- Continue irrigation during transport to a medical professional. This can be accomplished by having a portable eyewash unit located next to the permanent eyewash fountain. Continued irrigation is important because some chemicals, in viscous or powdered form, may continue to act for a period of time.
- Never work in the laboratory alone. You may be blinded and cannot help yourself. Table 4.28 lists the chemicals that frequently cause severe eye damage.

4.6.9 COMPRESSED GAS AND HANDLING GAS CYLINDERS[24]

4.6.9 A COMPRESSED GAS

Compressed gas cylinders can be extremely dangerous in the laboratory if not properly handled. A damaged cylinder has the capacity to jet away through brick walls, fly through the air, spin, or ricochet with the speed of a dragster. A standard oxygen cylinder may have the capacity of 244 cubic feet at 2200 pounds of pressure per square inch. The safe handling and use of these cylinders cannot be overstated!

All cylinders containing compressed gases such as oxygen, irrespective of whether they are flammable, should comply with specifications and should be maintained in accordance with regulations of the US Department of Transportation.

4.6.9 B HANDLING COMPRESSED GAS CYLINDERS

- Always check cylinders for contents before accepting shipment or connection.
- Transport cylinders with a dolly or hand truck to which the cylinder is secured.
- Secure the cylinder in place using a strap or chain support around the upper one-third of the cylinder body even when the cylinder is empty. Never leave a gas cylinder standing alone without secure support.
- Valve cap must be left in place until the cylinder is ready to be used. An unprotected valve can be damaged or even snapped off, unleashing the power of the cylinder through an opening no larger than a lead pencil.
- When connecting the regulator and hose, never force threads on the connection. If the regulator does not thread easily, something is wrong.
- The cylinder valve must be opened slowly, with the face of the gauge on the regulator pointed away from the face.

Table 4.27   CHEMICALS THAT MAY CAUSE SEVERE EYE DAMAGE

Acetic acid	Magnesium hydroxide
Ammonia	Potassium hydroxide
Calcium hydroxide	Sodium hydroxide
Chromic acids	Sulfur dioxide
Hydrochloric acid	Sulfuric acid
Hydrofluoric acid	

- Regulators, fittings, or gauges must not be lubricated with oil or any flammable substance.
- To avoid negative pressure build up in the tank, disconnect the hose or regulator, shut off the valve, and replace the cap before the tank is completely empty. Label the cylinder "empty."
- Cylinders must never be used as a "rack" for draping coats, masks, or face shields.

4.6.10 MAINTENANCE AND USE OF REFRIGERATORS[3,11]

Appropriate use of refrigerators in the laboratory is essential for the health and safety of laboratory personnel. The following stringent procedures must be implemented and maintained for safe use of refrigerators.

- Refrigerators must never be used for the storage of food or beverages.
- Personnel must avoid direct inhalation of refrigerator atmospheres. Because there is almost never an adequate ventilating device for the interior of refrigerators, the atmosphere in the refrigerator may contain a mixture of air combined with the vapor from flammable or toxic substances.
- There must be no source of electrical sparks within the refrigerator compartment.
- Modification of refrigerator units include removing any interior light that is activated by a switch mounted on the door frame; moving the contacts of the thermostat controlling the temperature to a position outside the refrigerated compartment; and removing the contacts for any thermostat present that controls fans within the refrigerated compartment to the outside of the refrigerated compartment. An alternative to modification is to place a prominent sign warning against storage of flammable substances within the unit.
- Where appropriate, purchase a unit that has been designated for "flammable storage" by the manufacturer.
- "Frost-free" refrigerators are not appropriate for laboratories because of modification problems. Drain tubes or holes direct water (and any flammable material present) to areas adjacent to the compressor and present a spark hazard.
- Refrigerators should be positioned against fire-resistant walls, have heavy-duty cords, and be protected by their own circuit breaker.
- Uncapped containers are not permitted in refrigerators.
- Containers capped with aluminum foil, corks, corks wrapped in aluminum foil, or glass stoppers are not permitted.
- Potentially explosive or highly toxic substances in laboratory refrigerators are discouraged. Prominent warning signs are displayed on the outside of the unit. Laboratories using such materials should purchase and use an explosion-proof refrigerator.
- Scheduled inventory and disposal of outdated or unnecessary materials must be maintained. Dispose of any materials that are not essential immediately.
- Storage of some reagents is best accomplished by refrigeration. Refrigeration of certain laboratory reagents refers to refrigeration of materials at temperatures between 4°C and 10°C. The best way to measure a refrigerator temperature is by keeping the thermometer in a clear glass bottle filled with water. The thermometer will be stable when read through the glass. Calibration and temperature should be documented at regular intervals using recording charts attached to the unit itself for easy access. Refrigerators and freezers are essential instrumentation in the laboratory. Stringent guidelines for use and maintenance of these instruments must be maintained.

4.6.11 MICROWAVE OVEN USE IN THE LABORATORY[25]

Microwave ovens have become prominent laboratory instrumentation and as standard equipment used in today's laboratory, they must be included in any comprehensive quality control program. Procedures for inspection, maintenance, and operation of the microwave oven should be included in the laboratory procedure manual.

4.6.11 A POTENTIAL HEALTH HAZARDS

The issue of health hazards arising from the use of "household" microwave units in laboratories is not unwarranted.[26] Several points must be addressed when operating a "household-type" microwave in the laboratory. These potential hazards include the following:

- Airborne concentrations of formalin vapors may be increased when using the microwave oven for fixation purposes (vapor concentration may well exceed the allowable PEL).
- Unvented oven chambers may release concentrated vapors when door is opened. (Chamber ventilation systems prevent buildup of toxic or flammable vapors and any vented air from the oven should be passed through the laboratory ventilation system or charcoal filter, or the oven should be enclosed in a hood.)
- Procedures using alcohols and xylene are flammable and potentially volatile. Potential ignition of volatile solution vapors may occur by a spark (switch) that turns off the magnetron when the door is opened (unless switch is explosion-proof).
- Solvent vapors may cause deterioration of door gaskets (if present) resulting in radiation leakage.

4.6.11 B CONTROL OF POTENTIAL HEALTH HAZARDS

Because of the aforementioned potential hazards, microwave units have been developed for laboratory use. These units are costly and for laboratories that use the nonlaboratory (household) units, some solutions are proposed to address these problems.[25]

- The use of zip-type bags, particularly those made for biological purposes, or at least, freezer-weight kitchen types, can be used to contain the fumes created when solutions are heated. (Thinner gauge bags will melt in the oven.) By enclosing the container in a completely sealed bag, fumes are contained.
- After heating, the container in the bag is taken to a fume hood and safely opened, reducing exposure to the technologist.
- Enclosing containers in bags also contains any spills that might occur, protecting the technologist from solution contact and preserving the surface of the oven interior.
- Minimization of the amount of solution used for many procedures, such as the use of microcontainers in place of coplin jars, further reduces the amount of vapor concentrations that may be produced.
- Control of volatile solutions is accomplished by quality control calibration of the oven, knowledge of boiling points of solvents, and controlled heating of such solutions when microwaved.
- The nonlaboratory or household microwave ovens manufactured currently do not have rubber-type gaskets at the door edge. If the oven does have a gasket, a routine inspection by a radiation safety officer should be able to detect if the gasket is no longer sealing the door properly.

- (c)(ii) "Microwave ovens shall be in compliance with the power density limits if the maximum reading obtained at the location of the greatest radiation emission, taking into account all measurement errors and uncertainties, does not exceed the limit specified in paragraph (c) (i) (shall not exceed 10 mW/cm^2 at any point 5 cm or more from the external surface of the oven) of this section when the emission is measured through at least on stirrer cycle."
- (c)(iii) "Measurement shall be made with the microwave oven operating at its maximum output and containing a load of 275±5 mL of tap water initially at 20±5°C placed within the cavity at the center of the load-carrying surface provided by the manufacturer. The water container shall be a low form 600-mL beaker having an inside diameter of approximately 8.5 cm and made of an electrically nonconductive material such as glass or plastic."

(21 CFR, Parts 800-1299, Food and Drugs, April 1, 1992)

It may be appropriate to place a warning label on microwave ovens. Figure 4.12 is an example of label precautions for safe operation.

Microwave regulation seems to be a "gray" area in laboratory safety, without clearly defined responsibilities of the laboratory personnel. Most regulations appear to be written with regard to the manufacturer's responsibilities. However, in the interest of good laboratory safety programs, all instruments used in the laboratory should be inspected regularly and have a standard schedule of maintenance. This includes the microwave oven. Figure 4.13 is an example of a chart used by radiation safety officers to determine microwave oven safety and integrity. A chart can be used to determine the temperature of a given amount of solution, heated at different times and different power settings (Figure 4.14). By demonstrating the final temperature of a given amount of solution, either aqueous or alcoholic, by the

---

Figure 4.12   WARNING LABEL ON MICROWAVE OVENS

Caution: Microwave oven in use

Precaution: avoid possible exposure to excessive microwave energy.

Do not operate this oven if:

There is an object caught in the door.

Door does not close properly.

Damaged door, hinge, latch, or seal.

Do not use any metal in oven.

Do not allow buildup of chemical or stain residue in oven chamber.

NOTE: This instrument is inspected regularly for radiation safety.

Figure 4.13   MICROWAVE OVEN SURVEY DATA SHEET[4]

Date _____

Department _____   Responsible Person _____

Location of Unit _____   Serial/ID # _____

Survey Instrument _____   Control Limit[1] _____ 10mW/cm^2

Inspection Checklist   **Yes   No   N/A**

1. Warning sign for radio frequency radiation posted. _____

2. Additional information or precautions included in the lower portion of the triangle. _____

3. Safety interlocks prevent the oven from operating if the door is opened.[2] _____

4. Additional warning sign posted at the entrance or in the vicinity of the oven. _____

5. Ovens are inspected periodically to insure proper operation. _____

6. Ovens are maintained in a sanitary condition. _____

Measurements: All measurements are taken at a distance of 5cm from the surface with 275ml of H_2O as load.

Door Closed
Readings mW/cm^2

1. ___ 2. ___ 3. ___

4. ___ 5. ___ 6. ___

7. ___ 8. ___ 9. ___

Max. reading____mW/cm^2

Interlock Test
Readings mW/cm^2

1. ____ 2. ___ 3. ___

4. ____ 5. ___ 6. ___

7. ____ 8. ___ 9. ___

Max. reading____mW/cm^2

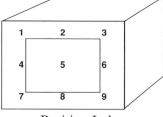

Position Index

Surveyed by_____

[1] 29CFR, Section 1910.97

[2] "Procedures for Field Testing Microwave Ovens," Bureau of Radiological Health, Nov. 1972, pg. 2.

Figure 4.14   MICROWAVE TEMPERATURE QUALITY CONTROL SHEET FOR AQUEOUS/ALCOHOLIC SOLUTIONS (CIRCLE ONE)

	Temperature (°C)									
Power	HI	90	80	70	60	50	40	30	20	10
10										
15										
20										
25										
30										
35										
40										
45										
50										
55										

Date Reviewed

_____

_____

_____

_____

_____

Technologist

_____

_____

_____

_____

power setting and seconds of heating, control of volatile solutions can be accomplished.

The Occupational Exposures to Hazardous Chemicals in Laboratories Standard, with its mandate for a chemical hygiene plan, is certainly one of the most significant regulations to have an impact on the laboratory environment. By the very nature of laboratory science, the highly complex involvement of chemicals is fundamental to this profession. Detailed and supplemental information has been included in this chapter to assist readers in developing their facility's chemical hygiene plan. It should be understood that additional, updated, and new information, particularly in the areas of chemical and dye hazards, is constantly being presented. Changes or amendments in the standard itself may also occur. It is important that the laboratorian keep abreast of these new developments and respond correspondingly.

4.7 REFERENCES

1. Montgomery L. *A Chemical Hygiene Plan for Occupational Exposures to Hazardous Chemicals in Laboratories, Education and Training Manual.* Baton Rouge, La: National Society for Histotechnology; 1990.
2. CFR 1910.1450. *Federal Register.* May 31, 1990;55(21):3300-3334.
3. Committee on Hazardous Substances in the Laboratory, National Research Council. *Prudent Practices for Handling Hazardous Chemicals in Laboratories.* Washington, DC: National Academy Press; 1981
4. Montgomery L. *Understanding the Right-to-Know Law, Education and Training Manual.* Baton Rouge, La: Louisiana State University School of Veterinary Medicine; 1988.
5. National Training Institute. *Instruction and Training Materials.* Washington, DC: Office of Training and Education, Occupational Safety and Health Administration; 1991.
6. Montgomery L. *Hazardous Chemicals in Laboratories.* Presented at the Conference on Histologic Technique; San Jose, Costa Rica; January 23, 1990.
7. Crookham J, Dapson D. *Hazardous Chemicals in Histopathology Laboratories.* 2nd ed. Battle Creek, Mich: Anatech Ltd; 1991.
8. Sharry J, ed. *Life Safety Handbook.* Boston, Mass: National Fire Protection Association; 1986.
9. American Chemical Society. *Less is Better, Laboratory Chemical Management for Waste Reduction.* Washington, DC: American Chemical Society Press; 1985.
10. Montgomery L. Decontamination of potentially infectious spills. *Tech Sample.* 1993;HT-1.
11. Farr K, ed. *Handbook of Laboratory Safety.* 3rd ed. Boston, Mass: CRC Press; 1991.
12. Stevens A. Finding and correcting flammable liquids hazards in the laboratory. *Am Lab.* 1990;22(10).
13. Montgomery L. *Hazardous Chemicals in the Electron Microscopy Laboratory.* Presented at the Electron Microscopy Society of American Meeting; Biloxi, Miss; 1989.
14. Montgomery L. Embedding media: an overview of hazards and safe handling. *Electron Micros Soc Am Bull.* May 1989;19(1):830-837.
15. Montgomery L. Report of health hazards of methacrylate and other plastics as embedding media: a project of the National Society for Histotechnology Health and Safety Committee. *J Histotechnol.* June 1989;12(2):143-144.
16. Center for Devices and Radiological Health (HFZ-30), Food and Drug Administration. Medical alert issued on allergic reactions to latex-containing medical devices. *Med Devices Bull.* April 1992.
17. Montgomery L. A review of the use of picric acid. *NSH in Action.* 1993.
18. Sheehan D, Hrapchak B. *Theory and Practice of Histotechnology.* 2nd ed. St Louis, Mo: CV Mosby Co; 1980.
19. Montgomery L. Tales of mercury poisoning. *LSH Network.* May 1994;12(2).
20. Montgomery L. Stop the insanity: use of mercury compounds must stop. *NSH in Action.* February 1994;21(1).
21. Ashbrook P. *Mercury: Chemical Health and Safety.* Washington, DC: American Chemical Society; 1994.
22. Crookham J, Dapson R. Drain disposal of laboratory chemicals. *Lableader Tech Bull.* Spring 1992:2,4,7.
23. Burns F. Prompt irrigation of chemical eye injuries may avert severe damage. *Occup Health Saf.* April 1989.
24. Klein B, ed. *Healthcare Facilities Handbook.* Boston, Mass: National Fire Protection Agency; 1986.
25. Crowder C. *Microwave and Conventional Procedures: A Manual of Histologic Techniques.* 2nd ed. Baton Rouge, La: Louisiana State University School of Veterinary Medicine; 1991.
26. Dapson R. Hidden hazards of the microwave oven in pathology. *Anatech Ltd Tech Bull.* 1989.

4.7.1   ADDITIONAL READINGS

Armour MA. *Hazardous Chemicals and Disposal Guide*. Boca Raton, Fla: CRC Press; 1991.

Asiedu S. Incompatible chemicals: an issue to consider, histologic. *Miles Inc Tech Bull*. November 1983;13.

Campbell S. A new look for the MSDS. *Occup Health Saf*. March 1992:62-65.

Cohen O. *Laboratory Design*. Washington, DC: American Chemical Society; 1987.

Collins G. *Systematic Approach for Safety Designing a Chemical Surety Material Laboratory*. Washington, DC: American Chemical Society; 1987.

Duetsch C. Safety standards and laboratory procedures for exposure to chemicals. *Lab Med*. 1992;23.

Gosta Axelsson C, Rylander R. Exposure to solvents and outcome of pregnancy in university laboratory employees. *Br J Industrial Med*. 1984;41:305-312.

Hembee D. News focus: high-tech hazards. *Ms*. March 1986:79-82.

Karcher R. Is Your Chemical Hygiene Plan OSHA-Proof? *Med Lab Observer*. July 1992:29-30,34-36.

Long J. Standard for MSDS in the offing. *Chem Engineering*. July 1991:7-11.

Mehne C. Quick and easy (protective equipment). *MT Today*. October 1993:12-14.

Mehne C. Positive protection. *MT Today*. October 1993:16-18.

National Fire Protection Agency. *Fire Protection for Laboratories Using Chemicals, National Fire Protection Agency Standard NFPA 45*. Batterymarch Park, Mass: National Fire Protection Agency; 1991.

Pedone M. Chemical hygiene plans: guidelines for compliance. *Am Lab*. June 1992:25-28.

Rekus J. Implementing chemical hygiene plans, focus of OSHA's new laboratory standard. *Occup Health Saf*. February 1990:52-59.

Ringo D, Read D. Glove material for handling epoxy resins. *J Electron Microsc Technique*. 1984;1:417-418.

Spake A. A new American nightmare? *Ms*. March 1986:35-42.

Stern A. Fire safety in the laboratory. *Lab Med*. 1993;24(5):275-277.

Tompkins N. Easier MSDS slides into view. *Occup Health Saf*. April 1992.

Tompkins N. Labor-supported committees advocate workers' right to understand the MSDS. *Occup Health Saf*. July 1991:23,24,47.

National Institute for Occupation Safety and Health, US Dept of Health, Education, and Welfare. *NIOSH Recommended Standard for Occupational Exposure to Xylene*. Washington, DC: National Institute for Occupation Safety and Health; 1975.

Vacca L. *Laboratory Manual of Histochemistry*. New York, NY: Raven Press; 1985.

Waxman M. New laboratory standard and chemical hygiene plan enhance workplace safety. *Occup Health Saf*. March 1992:20,25,66.

Weddington H. Legal risks in the histology laboratory. *J Histotechnol*. 1984;7:133-136.

Weintraub J. Caution: health hazards at work. *Vet Pract Med*. 1987:37-47.

Werely L. PPE selection for chemical use: looking beyond OSHA's guidelines. *Occup Health Saf*. November 1993:27-30.

Young J. A chemical hygiene plan: preparing, reviewing. *Industrial Hyg News*. March 1992.

Chapter 5

The Formaldehyde Standard

5.1 STATEMENT OF IMPLEMENTATION

The Occupational Safety and Health Administration (OSHA) passed the final ruling on May 27, 1992, with revisions becoming effective in 1993 for occupational exposure to formaldehyde.[1,2] The standard reduces the risk of exposure to workers from the hazardous effects of formaldehyde. It mandates that workplace exposure to formaldehyde be limited to a permissible exposure level (PEL) at or below 0.75 parts per million (ppm) and a short-term exposure limit (STEL) of 2.0 ppm per 15-minute exposure. The action level (AL) is 0.5 ppm.

Formaldehyde is an excellent preservative (fixative) for surgical and autopsy tissue. It is also an excellent germicide. Therefore, the obvious risk of exposure to workers in histology and pathology laboratories is apparent due to significant formaldehyde use. Because of frequent merging of laboratory functions, all areas and sections of the laboratory risk possible exposure to formaldehyde.

Even at relatively low levels (0.1 ppm), formaldehyde is an irritant to the skin and can cause tearing and irritation of the upper airways. Higher exposures are associated with cough, bronchial spasms, headaches, and dizziness. Dermatitis and asthma may also occur. Long-term exposure can result in pneumonitis and neuropsychiatric disorders including headache, irritability, and depression. The National Institute for Occupational Safety and Health (NIOSH) has labeled it a "potential human carcinogen."

A facility policy must be implemented to protect laboratory workers from health hazards associated with the use of formaldehyde in the laboratory. It is designed to identify actual and potential employee exposure, as well as to set forth responsibilities and activities to enhance employee safety. The formaldehyde exposure control plan, as well as the OSHA Formaldehyde Standard which requires that this policy be implemented, must be available to all personnel at all times during working hours. Figure 5.1 is an example of a statement of implementation.

Figure 5.1 STATEMENT OF IMPLEMENTATION

Effective Implementation Date _____

Laboratory Director_____

Chemical Hygiene Officer_____

Employee Signature _____

5.2 COMPLIANCE

5.2.1   BASIC STEPS
- Define job classifications and determine potential exposures for each worker or job classification.
- Monitor each worker initially, with respect to his or her exposure to formaldehyde.
- Develop and implement a formaldehyde control program that includes:
  - Engineering and work practice controls
  - Personal protective equipment (PPE) and respirator use
  - Housekeeping procedures
  - Emergency plan of action
  - Medical surveillance program with provisions for medical removal protection for workers suffering from formaldehyde exposure
  - Provisions for plan of action when exposure limits are exceeded
  - Hazard communication and labeling
  - Information and training program that includes (1) content of the standard and material safety data sheets (MSDSs); (2) potential health hazards of formaldehyde; (3) purpose and description of the medical surveillance program; (4) purpose, use, and limitations of PPE; (5) procedures handling spills, clean-up, and emergencies; (6) explanation of the importance of engineering and work practice controls in minimizing formaldehyde exposure; and (7) training to be given at least annually, with updates and refresher training as appropriate
  - Recordkeeping, including (1) exposure measurements and all monitoring documentation; (2) training and education; (3) respirator fit testing; and (4) medical surveillance and exposures
  - Disposal practices

5.2.2   GUIDELINES FOR COMPLIANCE

Only the essential requirements of the standard are outlined here. Before establishing a formaldehyde standard program it is recommended that a complete copy of the standard be reviewed.[1] For additional assistance regarding questions of the interpretation of the law itself or information concerning inspection compliance, refer to *Enforcement Procedures for Occupational Exposure to Formaldehyde*.[3] Single free copies are available by writing to OSHA Publications.

On December 2, 1987, OSHA issued the following statements concerning formaldehyde exposure:
- Formaldehyde is an irritant.
- Formaldehyde is a sensitizer.
- Formaldehyde is a potential human cancer hazard.

Histology, pathology, and anatomy laboratories were specifically mandated to comply in the same manner as do industrial manufacturers. Originally, the Formaldehyde Standard lowered the PEL from 3 ppm per 8-hour day to 1 ppm. However, on May 27, 1992, the standard was revised (Figure 5.2) and the PEL was lowered to 0.75 ppm. (Copies of the revised standard can be obtained from the General Printing Office, "New Order," PO Box 371954, Pittsburgh, PA 15260-7954. Enclose a check for $3.50 payable to Superintendent of Documents, or call 202-783-3236.)

Exposure limits are expressed as the maximum average full-shift exposure called the 8-hour time-weighted average (TWA) or as the 15-minute STEL concentration of formaldehyde in the air. The standard specifies a different set of requirements for each exposure limit, depending on the concentrations identified.[4] For instance:

- The AL is a concentration of formaldehyde of 0.5 ppm or more determined to be over the TWA.
- The PEL refers to the maximum allowable upper limit of exposure and in this standard the PEL is set at 0.75 ppm TWA.
- Short duration exposure (or STEL) is set by the standard at 2.0 ppm.

All employers are required to initially monitor exposures for each employee or job classification. Monitoring must reflect the exposure of the workers based on their job tasks, as determined by the employer.

An 8-hour day or 15-minute exposure must be measured depending on the circumstances of the work practice. It is important that each job classification be evaluated for potential exposure to formaldehyde and the anticipated exposure occurrences and exposure levels. In histology, each job assignment, such as changing the tissue processor, dissecting fixed specimens (trimming in tissues), transport and handling of tissue-filled cassettes, preparing formalin reagents, use of formalin in autopsies, preparing tissues for storage or disposal, etc, should be evaluated. The histology laboratory and the autopsy suite may have levels of formaldehyde that vary considerably, and only a limited number of workers may be exposed. Many such situations exist in the anatomic pathology section, and therefore the STEL may well represent the most accurate evaluation of formaldehyde exposure; however, in most cases, it will be necessary to monitor both the TWA and STEL levels. Figure 5.3 is a sample job classification monitoring form. Large institutions, where many workers may be exposed to formaldehyde, need to monitor at least 25% of the individuals on each shift in each job classification.[4]

Monitoring must be repeated if there is a change in procedure, personnel, or other circumstances that may result in exposure to formaldehyde. Regardless of exposure monitoring, if any worker complains of or exhibits signs and symptoms of formaldehyde toxicity, the worker must be monitored immediately. Monitoring may be performed by a laboratory employee using a hand-held infrared spectrophotometer or other direct reading instrumentation or air sampling chemical methods that meet OSHA specifications.[4] It is

---

Figure 5.2 REVISED (1992) EXPOSURE LIMITS

0.75 ppm per 8-hour day

2.0 ppm per 15 minutes short-term exposure limit

Action level remains at 0.5 ppm

---

very common for larger institutions or hospitals to contract the mandated formaldehyde monitoring to commercial firms that are equipped to do so. Make sure if you contract this portion of your program, that the company has proper credentials, adequate equipment, and appropriate references. It is important that all exposed workers be notified in writing of the monitoring results, and that they be given the opportunity to observe the monitoring procedure itself. (Many contract services comply with the written portion of this mandate by placing a sticker with all monitoring information in the appropriate area monitored for worker information and then providing an official report of monitoring results to the laboratory administration for proper filing.)

If mandated initial monitoring results are within the limits of an AL of 0.5 ppm and also within PEL and STEL limits (and if the monitoring methods and sampling are appropriate and correct), then monitoring does not have to be repeated unless there is a change in the procedures, processes, or other conditions that would indicate that an exposure might exist.[4,5]

If exposures are greater than 0.75 ppm, a medical surveillance program must be established.[1] (Consult the standard for complete details on this section of the law.)

An annual medical history questionnaire is to be completed by all workers with exposures over the AL (0.5 ppm) or the STEL, and depending on the evaluation of the reviewing

---

Figure 5.3 FORM FOR MONITORING SPECIFIC JOB CLASSIFICATION FUNCTIONS FOR FORMALDEHYDE EXPOSURE

Procedure/Process	Job Classification	Method	Time Monitored	Exposure	Date

physician, a physical examination may be required. (A questionnaire is provided within the standard.) Depending on the circumstances, this action can lead to annual medical checkups and further medical treatments. If exposures are greater than 0.75 ppm, monitoring must be done every 6 months; if the 15-minute level is greater than 2.0 ppm, monitoring must be done every year. In addition, if exposures are above 0.75 or 2 ppm, depending on the measured circumstances, the following requirements must be met.[3,5]

- Regulated areas must have warning signs.
- Exposures by engineering controls or by supplying full face respirators. The standard defines the type of respirator that is required for various levels of increasing exposure. For provisions regarding respirators, it is advisable to consult with a professional in respirator compliance. Considering the difficulties in securing proper respirators, fitting, and training in the use and maintenance of respirators, it is certainly prudent to correct any exposure problems utilizing engineering controls to reduce exposures.
- Safety showers and eyewash stations must be furnished.
- Personal protective equipment, such as gloves and goggles must be supplied.
- An emergency action (spill plan) must be established.

Other significant revisions in the Formaldehyde Standard (1992)[1] include the following:
- Evaluation for workers who develop medical problems due to exposure to formaldehyde, including:
- Medical evaluation at no expense to worker
- Evaluation of worker using "medical disease questionnaire"
- A determination by a physician as to whether a medical examination is necessary. If deemed necessary and an examination is undertaken, the physician must provide a written report to the employer and worker.
- A determination by a physician as to whether the worker is to be removed or restricted from work
- If a physician decides that no examination is necessary, a 2-week evaluation period is used to determine if signs or symptoms disappear with no treatment or with the use of PPE. If the symptoms or signs do not disappear, the worker is referred for medical examination and if work-related conditions are determined, transfer or removal from a particular job can be recommended.
- Medical removal protection for workers suffering from the irritant effects of formaldehyde exposure. This new rule defines the rights of those workers who have been removed, reclassified, suspended, or terminated from jobs. Failure to comply with this portion of the standard can result in serious legal liability problems. Records are to be maintained for 30 years.
- Employer must comply within 2 days of recommendation.
- Follow-up examination must be provided within 6 months to evaluate whether removal is permanent.
- If worker disagrees with findings or recommendations, he or she has the right to seek a second opinion (at no cost to worker if performed within 15 days of notification and worker notifies the employer and makes the appointment).
- If the two physicians disagree, a third physician, a specialist in occupational medicine, must evaluate the worker, performing any additional tests or examinations necessary.
- All physicians who examine or evaluate the worker must be supplied with (i) a copy of the Formaldehyde Standard, (ii) worker's job description, (iii) information concerning extent of exposure, and (iv) other relevant information such as PPE used.

- Expanding the one-time training requirement to annual training
- Omitting labeling requirements for formaldehyde-containing products that emit vapors in concentrations of less than 0.5 ppm. This new ruling has very little application to the anatomic pathology laboratory because concentrations of formaldehyde used in the laboratory are generally considerably higher (0.1 to 0.5 ppm).

5.2.3   METHODS OF COMPLIANCE[1,6]

5.2.3 A   ENGINEERING AND WORK PRACTICE CONTROLS

The standard requires employers to develop and implement engineering and work practice controls as the primary method of reducing and therefore minimizing employee exposure to formaldehyde. The employer shall apply these controls to reduce exposure limits to below the 0.75 ppm and, if unable to do so, will supplement these controls with respiratory protection.

5.2.3 B   RESPIRATORS AND PROTECTIVE CLOTHING AND EQUIPMENT

In the event that engineering controls are not sufficient or cannot achieve compliance levels with the PEL, the employer is required to provide and enforce the use of respiratory equipment to protect workers from exposure. Appropriate respiratory equipment and clothing must be furnished at no cost to the workers, and the employer must institute a respiratory protection program in accordance with the regulation (29 CFR 1910.134). Appropriate protective clothing (laboratory coats and aprons), gloves, face shields, and chemical protective goggles must be furnished. If face shields are used, chemical protective goggles are required to prevent formaldehyde from coming into contact with the eyes beneath the face shield.

5.2.3 C   HOUSEKEEPING

Employers are required to (1) institute a program for leak and spill detection; (2) perform preventive maintenance; (3) make provisions for spill containment and cleanup; (4) ensure that workers involved in cleaning up formaldehyde spills are trained and suitably equipped; and (5) label-sealed containers of formaldehyde.

5.2.3 D   EMERGENCIES

Employers must develop an emergency plan of action to minimize injury if there is any accident or spill involving formaldehyde. These procedures are performance-oriented and only need to be compatible with the facility and its use of formaldehyde.

5.2.3 E   MEDICAL SURVEILLANCE

Workers exposed to formaldehyde at or above the AL or STEL must undergo an annual medical screening and respond to an occupational disease questionnaire. Employers must make medical screening available to all persons exposed to formaldehyde in emergencies or who develop signs or symptoms that may be related to formaldehyde exposure. Any worker who is administered the questionnaire must be referred for additional testing if the physician reviewing the questionnaire believes such testing to be warranted. The physician must be supplied with (1) a copy of the Formaldehyde Standard, appendices, and revisions; (2) a copy of workers' job descriptions as they relate to formaldehyde (Figure 5.3); (3) the actual or representative exposure level; (4)

information on PPE used; (5) previous medical examination information; and (6) description of details surrounding circumstances (if emergency). A written opinion must be obtained from the physician, containing results of the examination and assessment of the employee's ability to work with formaldehyde without health impairment. The employer is required to retain records of medical examinations and must provide a copy of the physician's opinion to the worker within 15 days of receiving the opinion.

5.2.3 F HAZARD COMMUNICATION AND LABELING

The standard requires employers to comply with the general Hazard Communication Standard as it applies to labeling and the MSDS. The label must identify the hazardous chemical in a container, the manufacturer's name and address, state whether it is a potential cancer hazard, and include all potential hazards according to the Hazard Communication Standard. Labels must be present if the formaldehyde concentration of that solution exceeds 0.1% (Figure 5.4). That is, every container of formalin or formaldehyde-containing solution must have an appropriate warning label. The standard does not specify container size (volume of solution); therefore all and/or any container with formaldehyde that exceeds a 0.1% concentration must have a warning label. This includes the smallest biopsy bottle to the large specimen containers. Because of the extensive labeling and preparation procedures, many laboratories have resorted to buying commercially prepared, filled, and labeled specimen containers.

CAUTION: A frequently omitted requirement by manufacturers who are not in compliance, is a lot number and expiration date. If this information is not provided by a manufacturer, do not accept the material.[7] If you have containers of formalin without this information or the containers are filled by the laboratory (for in-house use or to send out to the clinic or doctor's office), then the laboratory must provide proper labels for the containers.

Material safety data sheets must be provided to those clinics or doctors' offices to which the laboratory supplies formalin bottles. (These off-site locations may need to institute their own formaldehyde training, monitoring programs, and emergency spill/leak procedures.[4])

NOTE: Solutions capable of emitting airborne concentrations less than 0.5 ppm do not have to have the potential cancer hazard warning. Most solutions in the laboratory have concentrations of 0.1 to 0.5 ppm.

5.2.3 G WORKER INFORMATION AND TRAINING

Employers must provide training at least annually to all personnel with the potential for formaldehyde exposure (Figure 5.5). All workers exposed to formaldehyde at levels of 0.1 ppm or higher on an 8-hour TWA basis are required to be included. The training material should include:
- The content of the Formaldehyde Standard and contents of the MSDS
- Description of the potential health hazards associated with formaldehyde
- The purpose and description of medical surveillance programs
- An explanation of safe work practices for limiting exposure to formaldehyde in each job classification
- The purpose, proper use of, and limitations of PPE
- Procedures for handling spills, cleanup procedures, and a review of emergency procedures
- An explanation of the importance of engineering and work practice controls in minimizing formaldehyde exposures

Figure 5.4 EXAMPLE OF A FORMALDEHYDE STANDARD ACCEPTABLE LABEL FORM

CAUTION: 10% FORMALIN

OSHA has determined that formaldehyde is an irritant, sensitizer,

and a potential human cancer hazard. May cause serious damage to the eyes

or blindness. Avoid skin contact, ingestion, and inhalation of fumes.

POISON!

Figure 5.5 RECORD OF TRAINING

Documentation of training in the Formaldehyde Standard:

Instructor _____ Department _____

(Name) _____ SS# _____ received _____

training in the Formaldehyde Standard. I have had an opportunity to ask questions of the instructor and understand the principles and goals of the Formaldehyde Standard.

Date _____ Employee Signature _____

Date _____ Instructor Signature _____

Additional training provided:

Date	Supervisor	Employee Signature

5.2.3 H   RECORDKEEPING

Employers must create and maintain accurate records of employee exposure (Figure 5.6). Workers must have access to these records and be notified if they have been exposed to substances above the PEL. Employers' records must include:

- Exposure measurements including date of monitoring; operation being monitored; method of sampling and analysis; all relevant sample data; protective devices worn; and names, job classification, social security number, and exposure estimates of employees represented by the monitoring
- Objective data used as a basis for exemptions from monitoring
- Medical surveillance
- Respirator fit testing

5.2.3 I   DISPOSAL PROBLEMS

Under the guidelines of the Formaldehyde Standard, requirements for the disposal of formaldehyde are not mandated because the law only covers issues dealing with worker safety. Disposal of formaldehyde and formaldehyde-containing solutions is the responsibility of the Environmental Protection Agency (EPA) and state and local authorities. There are some public-operated waterworks (POWs) that allow dumping of formaldehyde waste down the drain but there are just as many that do not. However, under the new EPA regulations, any facility dumping (formaldehyde) formalin down the drain must report it to the EPA.[7]

Figure 5.6 THE FORMALDEHYDE STANDARD DOCUMENTATION RECORD BASED ON DETERMINATION OF PERSONNEL/JOB CLASSIFICATION MONITORING

SS No.	Employee	Job Class	Exposure	Method Used	Monitored Time	Results

Solutions to the problems of formalin (formaldehyde) disposal may be forthcoming as our technology continues to expand. Some methods have already been developed and may warrant consideration, such as:

- Recycling formalin has now become a reality with some manufacturers having developed the instrumentation for the process. This relatively new technology is a sound alternative for formalin disposal and the economic benefits are apparent. Compared with the expense of having the formalin removed by a licensed hazardous waste service, recycling may be a highly effective alternative.
- Products for the neutralization or detoxification of formalin are now being supplied by various manufacturers. It is unwise to assume that these products render formalin safe to pour down the drain. Consult with your local officials. Beware of manufacturers who do not provide complete and detailed information concerning their products. Unfortunately, there are products on the market today that are simply not acceptable for solving the problem of formalin disposal.

5.3   FORMALDEHYDE CONTROL PLAN[8]

5.3.1   PURPOSE AND OBJECTIVES

The purpose and objectives of this plan are to maintain a system of inventory control, provide an effective method for reagent consumption, employ safe work practices to ensure a safe and healthy work environment, implement an emergency action plan for spills or leaks, and maintain an appropriate waste disposal system for control and removal of waste reagents. Figures 5.7 and 5.8 are forms required to be kept on record as part of an emergency plan.

5.3.2   STORAGE, SAFETY, EQUIPMENT, AND EMERGENCY ACTION

5.3.2 A   DISBURSEMENT AND USE

The formalin reagent is disbursed on a need basis in 1-gallon containers. Small amounts of formaldehyde may be maintained in laboratory areas for appropriate use in special stains and other established procedures. Under no circumstances are large quantities of formaldehyde to be maintained in the laboratory work area. Large containers (over 1 gallon) are to be returned to the storage area immediately after use.

Appropriate amounts of formalin (ie, 10% formaldehyde) may be maintained in the laboratory work areas as needed (ie, grossing areas). No substantial amounts of formalin are to be maintained in the laboratory work areas without significant reason, prior approval, and documentation of use (ie, mixing formalin solutions).

5.3.2 B   SAFETY EQUIPMENT AND PPE

Storage and laboratory use areas are to be equipped with a supply of appropriate gloves, chemical resistant face shields, safety glasses (with side shields), and respirators.

Safety emergency showers and eyewash stations are to be within immediate access to bulk storage and laboratory work areas.

5.3.2 C PERSONAL HYGIENE
Direct contact with the reagent or inhalation of vapors must be avoided. Exposed skin surfaces must be washed immediately if physical contact occurs. Clothes that become contaminated must immediately be removed and placed in a covered/sealed container for cleaning.

5.3.2 D SPILL OR LEAK CONTROL AND EMERGENCY ACTION
Figure 5.9 is an example of a form required as part of an emergency plan.

Figure 5.7 RESPONSIBLE PERSON

_____ (name and title)
_____ (location and phone)

is responsible for the acquisition, regulation, storage, monitoring, and enforcement of proper procedures for use, storage, and disposal of formaldehyde (formalin) reagents.

Figure 5.8 RECEIVING AND STORAGE

Bulk storage of formalin or formaldehyde is maintained in _____

The acceptable volume of this material is not to exceed_____

Figure 5.9 SPILL OR LEAK CONTROL AND EMERGENCY ACTION

_____ (name and title)
_____ (location and phone)

is the principal responsible individual to notify should any leak or spill occur.

5.3.2 E EMERGENCY ACTION FOR SPILL AND LEAKS

- Ask all nonessential personnel to leave the area in the event of a spill or leak.
- Wear appropriate PPE, gloves, full face shields, protective laboratory coat and apron, safety goggles, and respirators if appropriate.
- Contain the spill using a bag of absorbent on the spill site or absorb the spill with disposable paper towels as appropriate. Individual chemical containment may vary with the severity of the hazard. Consider specific chemical hazards including physical contact and inhalation of the chemical.
- Clean up the spill if appropriate. This procedure should be carried out by designated personnel trained in chemical spill procedures.
- Dispose of all waste material in appropriate sealed containers or bags for disposal services. (See also Table 4.3.)

5.4 REFERENCES

1. Occupational Safety and Health Administration. 29 CFR 1910.1048. *Workplace Exposure to Formaldehyde.* December 4, 1987;52:46291-46312.
2. Occupational Safety and Health Administration. 29 CFR 1910.1048. *Occupational Exposure to Formaldehyde: Final Rule.* May 27, 1992:22290-22328.
3. Occupational Safety and Health Administration. *Enforcement Procedures for Occupational Exposure to Formaldehyde.* Washington, DC: Occupational Safety and Health Administration; 1991. OSHA Instruction CPL 202.52.
4. Lott A, Greenblatt M. Formaldehyde regulations: what you need to know. *CAP Today.* April 1993.
5. Feldman A. *Special Report on the New OSHA Formaldehyde Standard.* Battle Creek, Mich: Anatech Ltd; 1988.
6. Bacharach Inc. *Technical Summary of OSHA's Final Rule on Workplace Exposure to Formaldehyde.* Pittsburgh, Pa: Bacharach Inc; 1987.
7. Crookham J, Dapson R. *Hazardous Chemicals in Histopathology Laboratories.* Battle Creek, Mich: Anatech Ltd; 1991.
8. Montgomery L. *The Formaldehyde Standard, Education and Training Manual.* Baton Rouge, La: Louisiana State University School of Veterinary Medicine; 1988.

5.4.1 ADDITIONAL READINGS

Goldman M, Stein A. Formaldehyde: Health effects, regulation and environmental control. *J Histotechnol.* March 1981;4:13-17.

Goldman M, Stein A. Toxic vapor control for automatic tissue processors. *J Histotechnol.* 1979:2:109-111.

Kilburn K. Neurobehavioral and respiratory symptoms of formaldehyde and xylene exposure in histology technicians. *Arch Environ Health.* 1985;40(4).

Kilburn K. Neurobehavioral effects of formaldehyde and solvents on histology technicians: repeated testing across time. *J Environ Res.* 1992;58:134-146.

Misiak P, Miceli J. Toxic effects of formaldehyde. *Lab Management.* 1986;24:134-146.

Chapter 6

The Bloodborne Pathogen Standard

6.1 Introduction to the Standard

Modern-day laboratory personnel are routinely made aware of the risk of exposure to bloodborne pathogens (BBP), and consequently safe techniques have been developed to minimize exposure to these pathogens. Blood and blood products are usually thought of as the vehicles for these BBPs. However, it must be remembered that other body fluids visibly contaminated by blood (ie, cerebrospinal fluid, amniotic fluid, urine, etc) and unfixed tissue can also be vehicles for BBPs.

Concerns about workplace exposure to two specific BBPs—human immunodeficiency virus (HIV) and hepatitis B virus (HBV), led the Occupational Safety and Health Administration (OSHA) to revise its exposure control regulations. Infection by HIV among health care workers has not significantly increased in the past few years; however, the reported incidence of *HBV* infection has risen dramatically by 37% among the general population from 1979 to 1989.[1]

Essentially the new OSHA standard (29 CFR 1910.1030), which became effective in March 1992, requires minimization of worker exposure to BBPs. The standard mandates that all laboratories establish stringent work practices and procedures that will ensure minimal exposure to these pathogens. Compliance with the standard was required by July 1992.[2]

OSHA's "Bloodborne Pathogen Standard" is a detailed and very specific document that will have a significant impact on the overall operation of our laboratories. Procedures and practices for compliance must be carefully determined on an individual laboratory basis. It is not the intent of this text to provide a lengthy and detailed examination of the standard but rather an overview of significant highlights of the standard. Readers are encouraged to obtain a copy of the standard for reference when establishing practices and procedures for their particular laboratories.

It should be emphasized that OSHA's BBP Standard, as their other regulations, is a performance-oriented one. This means that one compliance program may differ from other programs because of individual laboratory situations. As stated elsewhere, like chicken soup, there are hundreds of recipes, but in the end, they are all good soups.

In their efforts to comply, many safety managers, supervisors, and laboratory directors frequently bury themselves and their employees in a deluge of minute details because of their lack of understanding of the saying, "The main thing is to keep the main thing the main thing." The most important consideration when formulating your individual program should be the purpose—"employers shall provide a workplace free from recognized hazards" (OSHA Act, Section 5 A1)— rather than mere compliance with the regulations.[3]

6.2 Guidelines for Compliance[4,5]

The objective of the BBP Standard is to minimize worker exposure to BBPs in the workplace. The standard contains the following mandates for establishing an effective program to minimize these exposures.

6.2.1 TRAINING AND EDUCATION

An effective training and education program must be implemented (see also 6.11.10). The training program must include the following:
- The effective dates for compliance with the BBP standard and an explanation of the contents of the standard
- Training that is suitable to the audience
- An instructor who can answer questions or provide explanations regarding the training program. A simple impersonal video or sign-off document is not acceptable.
- Instruction given on the general epidemiology, modes of transmission, and symptoms of BBP disease with an emphasis on HIV- and HBV-related diseases

6.2.2 EXPOSURE CONTROL PLAN

Laboratories must establish an exposure control plan. All personnel must have knowledge of this plan and have access to the plan at all times.
- Task categories must be established to determine exposure potentials; all job descriptions must be listed, defining their potential for exposure. (See also 6.11.1.)
- HBV vaccinations must be made available to all personnel who may be exposed to potentially infectious material. (See also 6.11.7.)
- Procedures must be developed to evaluate the circumstances surrounding an exposure and to take appropriate action. Follow-up and evaluation procedures for exposure incidents are vital in preventing future incidents and are essential for compliance. (See also 6.11.8.)
- The plan must be reviewed and updated at least annually.

6.2.3 POSTEXPOSURE EVALUATION AND FOLLOW-UP

One of the most common violations in regulatory compliance is not establishing postexposure evaluation and follow-up procedures. Complete investigation, follow-up, and documentation of exposure incidents is an essential part of the laboratory health and safety programs. The importance of postexposure evaluation and follow-up procedures cannot be overemphasized. Figure 6.1 shows the guidelines for the evaluations and follow-ups.

If an exposure occurs, postexposure evaluation and follow-up that includes the following must be performed:
- Documentation of the route(s) of exposure and the circumstances related to the incident
- Identification of the source individual and, if possible, the status of the source individual. The blood of the source individual will be tested, after consent is obtained, for HIV/HBV infectivity.
- Results of the testing of the source individual should be made available to the exposed worker along with information on the applicable laws (including applicable local laws) and regulations concerning disclosure of the identity and infectivity of the source individual.
- Workers are offered the option of having their blood collected for testing of HIV/HBV infection. The blood sample should be maintained for 90 days to allow the worker to decide if the blood should be tested. Sample may be discarded if worker declines testing before 90 days.
- The worker should be offered postexposure prophylaxis in accordance with the recommendation of the US Public Health Service.

- The worker should be given appropriate counseling on precautions to be taken during the postexposure period. The worker must be given information on what potential illness to be alert for and to report any related experiences to appropriate personnel.

These postexposure evaluation and follow-up procedures and hepatitis B vaccination procedures are outlined in the OSHA Instruction CPL 2-2.44C (Office of Health Compliance Assistance).

6.2.4 RECORDS

Records of training, vaccinations, exposures, and follow-up evaluations must be maintained (Table 6.1). Records of *training* must be maintained for 3 years from the date of training and records of *exposures* must be maintained for at least the duration of employment plus 30 years.

6.2.5 METHODS OF COMPLIANCE

A control strategy with appropriate documentation must be established. Initially, a policy of universal precautions must be implemented (see 6.5). Universal precautions state that *all* human and other potentially infectious materials are treated as if they were infectious. The control strategy must include the following:

Figure 6.1 POSTEXPOSURE EVALUATION AND FOLLOW-UP GUIDELINES[12]

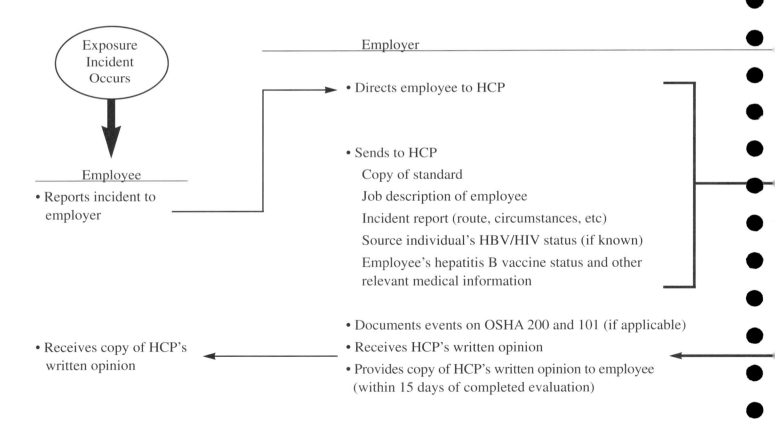

Exposure Incident Occurs

Employer
- Directs employee to HCP

- Sends to HCP
  Copy of standard
  Job description of employee
  Incident report (route, circumstances, etc)
  Source individual's HBV/HIV status (if known)
  Employee's hepatitis B vaccine status and other relevant medical information

Employee
- Reports incident to employer

- Documents events on OSHA 200 and 101 (if applicable)
- Receives copy of HCP's written opinion
- Receives HCP's written opinion
- Provides copy of HCP's written opinion to employee (within 15 days of completed evaluation)

OSHA Instruction CPL 2-2.44C Office of Health Compliance Assistance

- Engineering controls such as biological safety cabinets, autoclaves, puncture-resistant sharps containers, specially designed ventilation systems, and splash guards
- PPE, such as face shields, goggles, gloves, masks, gowns, and aprons. Determine the use of and policy for PPE, especially gloves, laboratory coats, goggles, and face shields. These policies will depend on the nature of the potential exposure (ie, masks in combination with eye protection devices). Surgical caps or hoods and shoe covers shall be worn in instances when gross contamination can be anticipated (ie, autopsies). All PPE shall be removed prior to leaving the work area.
- Work practices to minimize exposures include defining procedures to minimize splashing, spraying, and aerosolization; establishing systems of waste disposal in closable, leak-proof, labeled containers; developing procedures for the handling and disposal of sharps (needles must not be shared, bent, broken, or recapped by hand); establishing glassware handling procedures; establishing personal hygiene policies such as prohibiting eating, drinking, smoking, or application of cosmetics in the laboratory (even the use of lip balm or handling of contact lenses), and mandatory regular hand washing after removing gloves.
- Establishing housekeeping procedures with scheduled specific disinfecting practices, of bench tops, equipment, and other environmental surfaces. Procedures for safe handling of laundry must be established.

Health Care Professional (HCP)

C
O
N
F
I
D
E
N
T
I
A
L

- Evaluates exposure incident
- Arranges for testing of employee and source individual (if not already known)
- Notifies employee of results of all testing
- Provides counseling
- Provides postexposure prophylaxis
- Evaluates reported illnesses

- Sends (only) the HCP written opinion to employer:
  Documentation that employee was informed of evaluation results and the need for any further follow-up; and whether hepatitis B vaccine is indicated and if vaccine was received

- Establishing and implementing procedures for labels and signs as appropriate. All containers of blood or potentially infectious materials must be labeled. Appropriate labels should be placed on refrigerators, freezers, and waste containers. Red bags and red containers may be used in lieu of physical labeling. Labeling must display the biohazard symbol and the word "Biohazard." Labels and signs that are fluorescent orange or orange-red with blue, black, or green symbols or lettering are appropriate.

6.3 RESEARCH AND PRODUCTION LABORATORIES

For laboratories engaged in HIV and HBV research, additional requirements are mandated by the BBP Standard. Complete and detailed explanation of these requirements is found in the standard and all laboratories operating in this category should consult the standard for program compliance instruction. Requirements do not apply to clinical or diagnostic laboratories engaged solely in the analysis of blood, tissues, or organs. These requirements do, however, include all HIV and HBV research and production laboratories.

- Restricted access areas must be designated and labeled for:
  - Authorized personnel only
  - Special entry and exit procedures
  - Biohazard warning signs on access doors
- Waste handling procedures must be established including decontamination of waste prior to removal from the laboratory.
- PPE must be required, including:
  - Gowns, coats, gloves, and facial protection that must be worn in the work area
  - Protective equipment that must be removed before leaving the work area
  - Personal protective clothing that must be decontaminated before laundering
- Vacuum lines must be protected with liquid disinfectant traps and high efficiency particulate aerosol filters.
- All aspiration or injection procedures are performed using only needle-locking syringes or disposable syringe-needle units.
- A biosafety manual must be prepared and adopted and the program maintained.
- Biosafety cabinets are required. No work is to be done in open vessels or on open bench tops. Use of biological safety cabinets is enforced.
- Biological safety cabinets must be certified when first installed, whenever moved, and at least annually.

Table 6.1   DOCUMENTS AND RECORDS MAINTAINED

Records of personnel training (initial, updated, and annual)

Records of job classification/job description and exposure categories

Records of exposures, illnesses, and injuries

Records of postexposure, postillness, or postinjury follow-up and investigation

Records of medical surveillance and health care professional consultations

Records of hepatitis B vaccination or declination

6.4 Veterinary and Animal Research Laboratories

Personnel employed by veterinary or animal research laboratories may face certain risks that must be addressed. Frequently, veterinary and animal research laboratories conduct studies involving animal models of disease in which human pathogens are introduced. These studies may pose a direct hazard to individuals working with them. It is important to understand that appropriate protocol and safe laboratory practice are essential for the health and safety of veterinary and research personnel. Stringent guidelines should be observed for handling and disposal of specimens. As in all laboratory environments, cleanliness must be an essential part of the health and safety program.

6.4.1   ANIMAL TISSUE HAZARDOUS TO LABORATORY PERSONNEL[6]

- *Anthrax*: Acquired by man through contact with contaminated wool or other animal products or by inhalation of airborne spores
- *Brucellosis*: A generalized infection in man involving primarily the reticuloendothelial system
- *Rabies*: Fatal infectious viral disease of the central nervous system
- *Mad Cow Disease (Bovine Spongiform Encephalopathy)*: Related to scrapie, has demonstrated transference from sheep to cows and from cows to cats and dogs. Symptoms are similar to those of Creutzfeldt-Jakob disease (CJD). Its hazard to humans remains undetermined.
- Animals colonized or infected with noncommensals that are pathogenic to humans, such as choriolymphocytic meningitis virus carried by hamsters, simian immunodeficiency virus which infects primates, and mycobacteria
- Animals inoculated with human cell lines that may be infected with known human pathogens such as hepatitis or HIV or unknown human pathogens
- Agents that do not normally cause any pathogenic effects in the animal may be pathogenic to humans, such as toxoplasmosis carried by cats, Q fever carried by monkeys, or leprosy carried by armadillos
- *Animal Models of Human Disease:* Studies in which human pathogens such as *Salmonella* or *Shigella* have been introduced into rodents and other host animals (fish, primates, cats, and dogs)
- Various fungal agents, such as *Cryptococcus* or *Aspergillus,* which may be harbored in dirty drains, animal waste or debris, or air conditioning ducts

6.5 Universal Blood and Body Substance Precautions[7]

All human blood and body fluids are considered to be infectious; therefore, universal blood and body substance precautions are an important method of infection control. Significantly, barrier equipment is used to protect the health worker. Such barriers include gloves, gowns, waterproof aprons, masks, and protective face and eyewear.

All body substances such as respiratory secretions, feces, oral secretions, urine, and draining wounds may have organisms present that transmit disease.

Workers may incur risk each time they are exposed to blood/body substances. Any exposure may result in an infection and subsequent illness or death. Since it is possible to become infected from a single exposure, exposures must be prevented whenever possible.

6.5.1 MINIMUM REQUIREMENTS

Minimum requirements recommended during controlled situations to protect the health care worker from potentially infectious agents are not all inclusive, so judgment is required on the part of the worker to assess the need for additional barrier protection in less controlled situations. Frequent handwashing should be mandatory when performing all laboratory functions. Use of gloves is necessary in the performance of duties in which contamination is possible. Likewise, use of laboratory coats, gowns, aprons, and face protections is essential to prevent contamination. The use of hoods and personal respirators may be necessary wherever aerosolization of potentially infectious materials is anticipated.

6.5.2 STANDARD OPERATING PROCEDURES

- All specimens of blood and body fluids should be put in well-constructed containers with secure ties or seals to prevent leaking during transport. Care should be taken when collecting each specimen to avoid contaminating the outside of the container or the request slip accompanying the specimen. Contaminated specimen containers should be placed in a secondary container (double-bagged). Contaminated request slips should be reissued and the contaminated form disposed of appropriately.
- All persons processing bloody body fluid or tissue specimens should wear gloves. Persons with cuts or abrasions must use appropriate bandage coverings. Similarly, persons with dermatitis must not be exposed to potentially infectious materials.
- Gloves should be changed and hands washed after completion of specimen handling.
- For routine procedures such as histologic and pathologic studies or bacterial culturing, a biological safety cabinet is not necessary. However, biological safety cabinets (Class I or II) should be used whenever procedures are conducted that have a high potential for generating droplets. These include activities such as blending, sonicating, and vigorous mixing.
- Mechanical pipetting devices should be used for manipulating all liquids in the laboratory. Mouth pipetting must not be done.
- Use of needles and syringes should be limited to situations in which there is no alternative. No needles are to be recapped by hand, bent prior to disposal, or in any other manner handled unnecessarily.
- Contaminated materials/equipment used in laboratory tests should be decontaminated before processing or placed in bags and disposed of in an appropriate manner.
- Scientific equipment that has been contaminated with blood or other body fluids should be decontaminated and cleaned before being stored, repaired, or transported to other sections or manufacturers.
- All linen—towels, drapes, and laboratory coats—are considered contaminated and shall be handled as little as possible. These items are to be bagged or placed in hampers at the location of use in impervious bags and sorting or rinsing is to be avoided.
- *Cleaning and Disinfecting*: All equipment and environmental and work surfaces shall be properly cleaned and disinfected after contact with blood or body fluids. Work surfaces shall be decontaminated with disinfectant after completion of procedures when surfaces are overtly contaminated, immediately after any blood or body fluid spill, and at the end of work activities for the day. Protective coverings such as plastic wrap, aluminum foil, or imperviously backed absorbent paper may be used to cover equipment and environmental surfaces. These coverings shall be removed at the end of the work shift or when they become overtly contaminated.
- *Cleaning Blood and Body Fluid Spills*: Blood and body fluid spills shall be cleaned

promptly by using fresh solution of 10% household bleach or other appropriate disinfectant. Waste should be placed in plastic-lined infectious waste receptacles. Broken glass or other bits of material shall be picked up using forceps or other mechanical means such as a brush and dust pan.

- Telephones, computer stations, and/or other similar instrumentation shall be designated as either "clean" or "dirty"(contaminated). Depending on their use, appropriate work procedures are determined; for instance, if clean telephones are answered with gloves on, the receiver should be protected with a paper towel.

Table 6.2 lists the essential dos and don'ts in handling blood and body fluid spills.[8]

6.5.3 HANDWASHING

Handwashing is the single most important means of preventing infection and must be practiced before and after contact with patients or laboratory specimens and may be necessary during certain situations or procedures. Hands and other skin surfaces must be washed immediately and thoroughly if contaminated with blood or other body fluids. Always wash hands after removal of gloves.

Hands and other exposed skin areas should be washed:
- Whenever there is visible contamination with blood or body fluids
- After the completion of work and before leaving the laboratory area
- After removing gloves
- Before eating, drinking, smoking, applying makeup, changing contact lenses, and using lavatory facilities

Table 6.2   BLOOD AND BODY FLUID SPILL PROCEDURE[8]

1. Wear gloves and laboratory coat, face protection if appropriate.

2. Do not remove any glass or other sharp objects with hands. Use a rigid cardboard as a "pusher"and "receiver." Discard in puncture-resistant biohazard container.

3. Absorb the spill with disposable materials such as paper towels or commercial absorbent material.

4. Clean all visibly spilled material using a detergent. Common household detergent will do.

5. Disinfect the spill site with a 1:10 solution of bleach (sodium hypochlorite). Flood spill site or wipe down the spill site with disinfectant-soaked paper towels.

6. Absorb disinfectant with paper towels, dry area, or allow to air dry.

7. Discard all materials in the biohazard container.

8. Wash hands and exposed skin areas thoroughly.

OR   1. Wear gloves and laboratory coat, face protection if appropriate.

2. Use commercial spill kit according to kit instructions.

3. Discard all materials in biohazard container.

4. Wash hands and exposed skin areas thoroughly.

- Before all other activities that entail hand contact with mucous membranes, eyes, or breaks in the skin.

Washing with soap and water is recommended. Any standard detergent may be used. Hand-wipe towelettes and cleaning foams do not provide appropriate dilution and detergent action and are not followed by rinsing. Therefore, they are not recommended except in field conditions where water is not available. No additional benefit has been established for washing with antiseptic soaps or antiseptics. Products that may disrupt skin integrity should not be used. Using a moisturizing hand cream may reduce skin irritation caused by frequent handwashing.

Facilities for handwashing should be provided in each laboratory area. The handwashing area should be separate from those used for washing equipment or for waste disposal and should be clearly designated as a "clean sink" or "handwashing" area.

Figure 6.2 is a handwashing sign that may be posted in laboratories.

6.5.4 PROTECTIVE BARRIERS

6.5.4 A GLOVES

Wear gloves whenever touching blood and body fluids, mucous membranes, or nonintact skin of all patients, and whenever handling items or surfaces soiled with blood or body fluids. Gloves should be changed after handling contaminated specimens. Disposable gloves should be replaced as soon as possible when visibly soiled, torn, punctured, or when their ability to function as a barrier is compromised. Gloves should not be washed or disinfected for reuse.

Gloves must be worn:
- By all laboratory personnel who anticipate contact with tissues; blood; serum; plasma; cerebrospinal fluid; vaginal secretions; semen; bronchopulmonary washings; synovial, pleural, peritoneal, amniotic, and pericardial fluids; breast milk; or other bodily material visibly contaminated with blood
- By all personnel when handling biohazard bagged material and visibly contaminated items or linen
- By personnel using equipment that is likely to be contaminated, such as a biological safety cabinet. These instruments must be labeled as biohazards and the use of gloves specified.
- Because HBV can be transferred from hands to laboratory surfaces and thus to other hands, gloves should be removed before handling telephones, uncontaminated laboratory equipment, doorknobs, etc. Alternatively, specific instruments, such as computer keyboards and telephones, may be specifically labeled as a biohazard and used only with gloves. Care must be taken not to use these marked ("dirty") instruments with ungloved hands.

Standard operating procedures for glove use include the following:
- Latex or vinyl gloves provide adequate barrier protection; however, latex is less likely to develop leaks during use. (See also Chapter 9.)
- Gloves made of thin latex or vinyl are not intended to provide protection from puncture wounds caused by sharp instruments.

Figure 6.2 A Handwashing Sign for the Laboratory

Handwashing is the best way to prevent the spread of infection...

PLEASE WASH YOUR HANDS

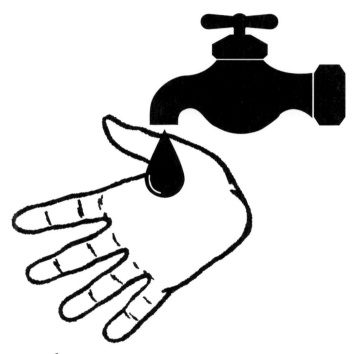

Handwashing procedure:

1. Use continuously running water.
2. Use a generous amount of soap.
3. Apply with vigorous contact on all surfaces of hands.
4. Wash hands for AT LEAST 10 seconds.
5. Clean under and around fingernails.
6. Rinse with your hands down, so that runoff goes into sink, and not down your arms.
7. Avoid splashing.
8. Dry well with paper towels.
9. Use a towel to turn the water off.
10. Discard the towels into a bag provided for that purpose.

- Gloves are intended to cover defects in the skin of the hands.
- Latex gloves are preferred because there is some evidence that a latex glove provides protection (a "wiping action") that diminishes the amount of blood or other material transmitted to a wound created by a needle.
- Single gloves protect the hands from contamination with blood and body fluids.
- Heavyweight utility gloves may be used during high risk activities such as dishwashing.
- Stainless steel mesh gloves protect against injury caused by large sharp edges such as knife blades.
- Double gloving is recommended during autopsies or other situations in which gross contamination of gloves may be anticipated.
- Gloves should be disposable (latex/vinyl) and changed frequently.
- Used gloves should be discarded in biohazard waste containers.
- Gloves should be examined for visible defects after donning and before commencing work.
- Gloves should be changed if they become visibly contaminated or if physical or chemical damage occurs.
- Gloves need not be changed during laboratory activities that routinely result in contaminated gloves (such as trimming tissue). However, gloves should be changed when these tasks are completed or a breach in the glove occurs.
- Aseptic technique should be used for donning and removing gloves.
- Do not wash or disinfect gloves for reuse.
- Use general purpose utility gloves, such as rubber household gloves, for house-keeping and decontamination procedures. Utility gloves may be decontaminated and reused but discarded if there is any evidence of damage or deterioration.

6.5.4 B   GOWNS OR LABORATORY COATS

Fluid-resistant clothing should be worn during procedures that are likely to generate splashing of blood or body fluids. Gowns, laboratory coats, or aprons should be worn if there is a potential for soiling clothes with blood or body fluids.

6.5.4 C   MASKS, PROTECTIVE EYEWEAR, AND/OR FULL-FACE SHIELDS

Protective face wear should be worn during procedures that are likely to generate splashes, sprays, splatters, droplets, or aerosols of blood or body fluids to prevent exposure of mucous membranes of the mouth, nose, and eyes. Full-face shields should be sufficient to cover the face to beneath the chin.

6.6   GUIDELINES FOR PERFORMING AUTOPSIES[5,7]

The operations of anatomic pathology laboratories have been dramatically affected by numerous guidelines, regulations, and other factors such as the availability of new protective devices and equipment to prevent injury and exposure to BBPs particularly HIV infection. Prevention of exposure to HIV, HBV, other bloodborne infections, and tuberculosis is of primary concern. Nowhere in the laboratory are precautions more essential than in the autopsy suite.

Autopsies should be performed using universal precautions (see also 6.5). Using guidelines provided by the Centers for Disease Control and Prevention, it is possible to perform autopsies under almost all conditions with minimal risk to personnel. Studies have demonstrated that HIV is clearly viable in the postmortem period (0 to 20 hours) during which most autopsies are performed.[9]

6.6.1 PERSONAL PROTECTIVE EQUIPMENT

The following PPE must be used for performing all autopsies (whether considered infectious or noninfectious):

- Scrub suits, not street clothing, to prevent particulate material from leaving the autopsy suite
- Long-sleeved disposable gowns made of fluid-impermeable plastic
- Hair and foot covers, goggles, face mask, and gloves
- Face shield covering entire face and neck. Various combinations of facial protection, but especially for the eyes, nose, and mouth
- Personal respirator under shield to prevent airborne contamination
- Double latex gloves covering cuff of clothing. Additional utility gloves over latex gloves. Stainless steel mesh gloves covered by latex gloves to reduce slippage, protect against scalpel, or bone puncture
- Fluid-proof foot covers or protective boots

6.6.2 PERSONNEL

6.6.2 A   SPECIAL TRAINING

Autopsy procedures require special training of personnel, particularly concerning accidental injury.

6.6.2 B   LIMITED NUMBER OF PARTICIPANTS

Limit the number of participants in autopsies to two or three workers—a prosector (contaminant contact) and an assistant/circulator—particularly when a case is known to be infectious. A "clean" circulator is especially recommended to handle cultures or other containers, answer the telephone, handle paperwork, and obtain instruments or equipment.

6.6.3 PROTOCOLS AND PROCEDURES

Procedures for performance of autopsies should be the same for cases considered infectious and those considered noninfectious. This establishes the standard for autopsy performance and eliminates unnecessary stress if a case is later found to be infectious.

- Modify all procedures to reduce splashing or avoid blind dissections.
- Single scalpel handle should be used by prosector to open skin. Disposable scalpels reduce the need to change blades.
- Use blunt-tipped scissors to perform autopsies.
- Leave all instruments and specimens on table until autopsy is complete; place in tray for transport and cleaning.
- Bone saws, wrapped in plastic, are used with vacuum attachments to reduce dispersal of dust or droplets. Vacuum attachments produce unfiltered exhaust and may be hard to decontaminate. Alternative methods may be developed such as a damp drape system. (See also 6.6.3 A.)

- Instruments are not to be transferred by hand, but placed on the table to be picked up by the other person.

6.6.3 A   REMOVAL OF THE BRAIN

The removal of the brain is a major concern. Sawing through the calvarium is especially dangerous. Hand saws are not recommended because of the high risk of injury. A vibrating saw is preferred, using clear plastic drapes placed over the head and neck area. There are a number of commercial autopsy drapes available today; however, laboratory personnel can design their own drapes, which work equally well. The main concern is to prevent aerosols or splashes. There are also commercial units now available that enclose the entire body and are completely self-contained with gloved arms, drainage plugs, and inlet ports for water or electrical lines. This type of unit might be especially useful in suspected cases of CJD. Once the autopsy is complete the unit is collapsed and the entire body can be placed in a body bag. This is particularly suitable for cremation where the entire unit is burned but other cases that require removal of the body from the bag might face a potential contamination problem.[9]

There are also suction units that can be attached to Stryker saws but these seem to provide limited protection from aerosolization. The air blowing out of the back of the unit is not filtered, and sterilization of these units is difficult. Aerosolization can be dramatically reduced by simply placing damp towels around the area. Irrigation of the area with water is also effective in reducing bone dust particles.

6.6.3 B   DELAYED DISSECTIONS

If possible, delay detailed dissections of tissues involving cases of known BBPs or tuberculosis, until the tissue specimen is completely fixed.

6.6.3 C   PHOTOGRAPHY

Prudent use of photography and the use of hand-held cameras are encouraged.
- Tissue specimen must be transported to the camera stand in a transport pan by the assistant.
- The prosector, after rinsing gloved hands, may arrange tissue specimen for photography.
- Only the assistant should handle the camera.
- Tissue specimen is returned to the table in the transport pan or is fixed.
- If a camera stand is used, it must be thoroughly decontaminated following use.

6.6.3 D   AUTOPSY AREA

- Designate as a "biohazard" area.
- Post biohazard warning signs at all entrances.
- Consider the entire area and all its contents as potentially infected.
- List individual hazards and required precautions on entrance signs.

6.6.3 E   DECONTAMINATION

Decontaminate the entire area—tables, contents, and floors—with appropriate germicide for any suspected contaminants such as HIV, CJD, and tuberculosis.

6.6.3 F COLLECTION OF SPECIMENS

- *Blood or Culture Material*: Needles are not to remain on the table. Follow universal precautions; containers are not to be held by hand when introducing specimens.
- *Tissue Specimens*: Tissues are placed in fixative while on the table; container exteriors are decontaminated before removal.
- *Unfixed Specimens*: Place in leak-proof containers; place in secondary container for transport; label as a biohazard; large sections must be "bread-loafed" prior to fixation for maximum fixation; minimize collection of unfixed tissue; double bag and label "biohazard"; incinerate immediately following examination or fix the tissue.

6.7 HANDLING AND TRANSPORT OF SURGICAL SPECIMENS

6.7.1 PERSONAL PROTECTIVE EQUIPMENT

- Aprons, gowns, and double gloves
- Facial protection if large or bloody specimen

6.7.2 CONTAINERS

- Screw top containers minimize splashing associated with "snap on" lids.
- Exterior of all specimen containers is considered contaminated.
- Primary containers (bottles or fixed tissue) must be placed in secondary leak-proof container.
- Requisition slip is kept uncontaminated in a separate plastic sleeve or bag.

6.7.3 IMPRINTS, CYTOLOGY, BONE MARROW, SMEARS

- All smears are to be considered contaminated until fixed in alcohol or formalin.
- Air-dried specimens are infectious for "a period of time" after preparation.

6.7.4 BODY FLUIDS

- Body fluids are considered extremely dangerous.
- Double gloves, gowns, aprons, and facial protection are necessary.
- Prepare specimens in safety box or biological cabinet if droplet dispersal is high.
- Safety centrifuge cups with caps are essential if airborne agents are suspected.

6.7.5 DECONTAMINATION

- Decontaminate surgical dissection area in a manner similar to the autopsy area. (See also 6.6.3 E.)
- Decontaminate exterior of specimen containers.

6.7.6 MATERIALS CONSIDERED NONINFECTIOUS

These include:
- Paraffin blocks.
- Coverslipped, fixed, and stained slides.

6.8 PROCEDURES FOR PROCESSING CJD TISSUE

An important part of any laboratory health and safety program is having established procedures for handling and processing of tissues suspected of being infected with Creutzfeldt-Jakob disease (CJD). The disease causes a slow progressive dementia of the central nervous system. Although CJD resembles two other diseases, kuru and scrapie, the transmissible agent of the disease demonstrates very unusual characteristics. The disease has a long incubation period, up to 8 years in some cases; it does not provoke an inflammatory reaction within the infected tissues; it has never been isolated; and importantly, it is resistant to routine paraffin processing. Treatment of tissue specimens having CJD with long sterilization at high temperatures or prolonged exposure to bleach has proven effective in deactivating the agent.[10]

Because of the rising incidence of AIDS and the increased awareness of other infectious diseases, technologists must address special attention to handling potentially infectious tissue in the laboratory. Precautions and procedures to safeguard personnel from the hazards of these diseases are an essential part of laboratory procedure manuals and are required for inspection agencies such as the College of American Pathologists. Procedures should include any suspected cases of CJD or any unexplained cases of encephalopathy in a patient.

Significant aspects of the disease include the following:
- CJD requires histologic examination of tissues for diagnosis.
- CJD is a progressively fatal disease of the central nervous system affecting one to two individuals per million per year worldwide.
- CJD is resistant to formalin fixation, alcohol dehydration, and paraffin embedding as well as to moderate temperature.
- Paraffin blocks and tissue sections containing CJD are potentially infectious.

6.8.1 EPIDEMIOLOGY AND MODES OF TRANSMISSION

- CJD has been categorized along with kuru, scrapie, and transmissible mink encephalopathy because these chronic brain infections exhibit similar unusual vacuolar encephalopathy. These conditions are referred to as transmissible spongiform encephalopathies.
- Patients with CJD exhibit progressive dementia including personality changes, abnormal electroencephalograms, and jerking motions. Neurologic findings may mimic other diseases such as Alzheimer's disease.
- Most patients are in their 60s; however, patients as young as 17 years have also been reported. Death occurs usually within 1 year of diagnosis.
- Biopsy or tissue section is essential for diagnosis of CJD. The agent responsible for this disease has never been satisfactorily isolated.

6.8.2   LABORATORY PRECAUTIONS

- Gloves are worn during all phases of handling tissue samples with CJD disease (or other unexplained cases involving encephalopathies).
- Tissue samples from autopsies and brain biopsies are examined grossly and dissected using special kits. All tissue samples are potentially infective but infectivity decreases peripherally in other organs and tissues.[11]
- Special color-coded tissue cassettes are reserved to indicate potentially infectious tissue of a significant nature such as CJD.
- Tissue samples left over after dissection are placed in formalin, double bagged, and appropriately tagged with an "infectious hazard" label. Some authors recommend a solution of phenolized formalin prepared by adding 15 g of phenol per 100 mL of neutral-buffered formalin.[11] This phenol-formalin fixation is thought to reduce the infectivity of the tissue so that handling of the tissue, as a practical matter, is risk free.[11]
- An entire brain should be immersed in phenol formalin for several weeks. Slicing the brain will enhance the process.
- An alternative method advocates prefixation in a solution of formic acid (95%) for 1 hour, transferred to formalin for 2 days, and then processed.[11]
- Specimens of CJD or unexplained encephalopathies are processed separately from routine tissues and sectioned on a microtome reserved for significantly hazardous tissues.
- Following each step of the procedure, the area is cleaned and sterilized using a 10% bleach solution.
- All materials used in the process such as the infectious tissue kit; trimmed wax from the microtomy process; waste sections of tissue, gauzes, towels, etc; and gloves are incinerated after use.
- Processing fluids from the tissue processor and stain solutions are placed in containers, appropriately labeled, and disposed of according to the institution's requirements. (Fluids and instruments can be steam-autoclaved for 1 hour at 132°C [15 psi] and then discarded normally. They must not be reused.[10])
- All instruments and equipment such as baskets from processors, forceps, and embedding molds must be soaked for 1 hour in a 10% bleach solution even though minor corrosion of the instruments will occur. Wash and rinse well.
- The exterior of the microtome is wiped with bleach and rinsed with water. Because the microtome is impossible to thoroughly disinfect it must always be considered infectious. Disposable blades are incinerated.

6.9   Guidelines for Safe Use and Maintenance of the Cryostat[12]

- Frozen sections are not performed unless necessary.
- Gloves must be worn.
- The entire contents of the cryostat are to be considered biohazardous.
- Tuberculocidal fixative (alcoholic formalin) must be used as follows:
    - 900 mL   50% ethyl alcohol
    - 100 mL   37% (full strength) formaldehyde

6.9.1 PPE REQUIRED

- Gloves (vinyl or latex) must be used for routine sectioning.
- Gloves (stainless steel mesh) should be worn when handling the microtome blade or cleaning/decontaminating the instrument.
- Full face shields should be used if splattering is likely.
- Laboratory gowns or coats with gloves covering the cuffs are required; arm sleeves are acceptable for use.

6.9.2 SPECIAL INSTRUCTIONS

Freezing propellants under pressure should not be used as they may cause splattering or droplets of infectious material.

If the specimen is suspected to be infected with HIV, HBV, or other BBPs or if the tissue is suspected of containing *Mycobacterium tuberculosis*, the cryostat must be defrosted and decontaminated immediately with tuberculocidal disinfectant.

The cryostat must be decontaminated immediately after routine use. All exposed internal and external surfaces of the unit should be wiped with 95% ethyl alcohol and allowed to air dry for 15 to 20 minutes. Any excess alcohol is dried off and the microtome lubricated as needed. The microtome blade holder and blade is removed from the microtome and soaked in a container of 95% ethyl alcohol. Similar action is used for disposable blade holders and blades. The disposable blades are discarded in a puncture-resistant container after they have been decontaminated.[13]

Complete defrosting and decontamination of the cryostat should be performed immediately after contamination by any known infectious material, before any maintenance service or transport of the unit to another location or facility. Decontamination of the cryostat is usually dealt with in the same manner as HIV decontamination; in most instances, these precautions are applicable to TB as well. However, the CDC recommends a 5% phenol–absolute alcohol solution for cleaning the interior of the cryostat as well as all contaminated paraphernalia. The NCCLS recommends a 10% formalin–50% ethanol fixative solution when *M tuberculosis* is suspected. It must be remembered that phenol is a hazardous chemical. Appropriate gloves and mask should be used when handling this material, and absorption through the skin or inhalation of fumes is to be avoided. However, there seems to be conflict between the use of phenol products and OSHA regulations. It is recommended that you check with your local agency or state regulations before introducing the use of any new product.

CAUTION: Because cuts of the hands are common and adequate decontamination of the cryostat is difficult, frozen sections should not be cut on unfixed tissue unless there is a pressing need. Only authorized personnel may use, maintain, or otherwise service this instrumentation (Figure 6.3).

6.10 RESPIRATORY PROTECTION[14,15]

Respiratory protection in the laboratory has been mandated by the OSHA Respiratory Protection Standard 29 CFR 1910.134 (1984). The promulgation by OSHA is currently undergoing revision and may be some time in coming because of the regulatory process.[14] Unfortunately, the standard has not been revised since 1984 and there have been dramatic advances in information regarding respiratory protection. The original standard does, however, provide guidelines for establishing a respiratory protection plan for the laboratory. Another, more current guideline and one that more clearly reflects the current state of technical knowledge in respiratory protection, is the ANSI Z88.2-1992 Practices for Respiratory Protection. The ANSI standard is a voluntary consensus standard that is, in many aspects, more strict in its guidelines than the OSHA standard.[15] It is, however, up to the individual developer of the facility respiratory protection plan to determine which set of guidelines to follow. It is suggested that copies of both guidelines be made available in the laboratory for reference to specific detailed information regarding respiratory protection. Many facilities find it prudent to consult professionals when establishing their respiratory protection programs.

6.10.1   OSHA RESPIRATORY PROTECTION STANDARD REQUIREMENTS

- Written standard operating procedures for respirator use
- Procedures and practices for program evaluation and review
- Methods for selection of respirators
- Training and education of personnel
- Fit testing for individuals likely to use respirators
- Inspection, cleaning, maintenance, and storage procedures
- Medical examination or consultation as appropriate
- Surveillance of appropriate respirator use
- Air quality standards
- Approved respirator types

6.10.2   PERSONNEL EDUCATION AND TRAINING REQUIREMENTS

- Sources of respiratory hazards
- Engineering and work practice controls
- Selection of respirator types
- Limitations of respirators
- Methods for use and individual fit checks
- Maintenance and storage of respirators
- Emergency situation procedures

Figure 6.3 Sample Form for Documenting Use and Maintenance of the Cryostat

Date	Case #	Procedure			Decontamination		Comment	Physican/Technician
		Fixed	Unfixed	Routine	Defrost			

6.10.3 USE AND MAINTENANCE OF RESPIRATORS

A number of regulations may require the use of respirators in the laboratory. Depending on the situation, whether chemical or biohazard, the selection of respirators must be specific for use. Chemical respirators require individual personal fittings. Many facilities find consulting specialists trained in respiratory requirements to be highly valuable. This is because they eliminate some of the confusion regarding respirator selection as well as provide appropriate training and individual fittings of respirators. There are, however, steps that all facilities may take regarding respirators, particularly in the area of biohazards.

Guidelines issued by the Centers for Disease Control and Prevention has issued the following guidelines[16]:

- The use of personal dust and mist respirators (NIOSH approved) is recommended if there is a possible exposure to *M tuberculosis* as during the autopsy procedure or when aerosols are produced (Table 6.3). Available as disposable or reusable types.
- Surgical masks protect the nose and mouth from the splattering and splashing of material but become saturated quickly and therefore are not recommended.
- Personal respirators should be covered with a full face shield if splattering is likely, as in autopsy procedures.

6.10.4 OSHA REQUIREMENTS FOR MAINTENANCE OF RESPIRATORS

"Respirators shall be cleaned and disinfected after each use." There are no clear OSHA- or NIOSH-defined standards for what constitutes regular or thorough cleaning or disinfecting of respirators. Laboratories must decide what constitutes proper maintenance to meet OSHA regulations and ensure that this maintenance does not damage the equipment.[17]

A number of methods have been used to clean respirators but most of them appear to inhibit effective use, create substantial damage, are unpleasant for use, and in fact, do not provide disinfecting results at all (Table 6.4). Use of quaternary ammonium is the most effective cleaning method for laboratory use. It is an excellent cleaner, disinfectant, and deodorizer. It is available in bulk concentrates, ready-to-use spray bottles, and prepackaged towelettes. With bulk concentrates, cleaning is easily accomplished by mixing the concentrate (according to instructions) with warm water, immersing the respirator in the solution for 2 minutes, rinsing with water thoroughly, and allowing to air dry. The respirator is then ready to store in a plastic zip-type bag. Be sure to document the cleaning by labeling the plastic bag with the date and initials of the responsible personnel. Store out of sunlight to prevent damage.

Table 6.3   LABORATORY PROCEDURES THAT MAY RESULT IN AEROSOLIZATION OF PARTICLES

Accidents, spills, or breakage	Lyophilization
Animal handling	Mixing, blending, stirring, grinding
Breaking ampules	Pipetting
Centrifugation	Powder handling
Clean-up, especially dry sweeping	Removing caps, stoppers, lids
Combustion	Size reduction, grinding, chipping
Heating, evaporation/condensation	Transfer operations
Injections using needles and syringes	Ultrasonic procedures

Table 6.4 UNSATISFACTORY METHODS FOR CLEANING RESPIRATORS[17]

CLEANER	REASON
Bleach	Attaches to and corrodes metals and certain fibers.
Soap and water	Does not disinfect.
Iodine	Strong aftersmell in the mask
Heat (for washing or drying)	Dries out rubber, may melt some parts; also must be stored out of sunlight for the same reason.
Alcohol	Towelettes good for disposable respirators but because alcohol evaporates rapidly, it is not considered a true disinfectant.
	Dipping in alcohol-saturated materials will disinfect but damage rubber or neoprene causing dry rot, cracking, or splitting.
	Silicon inhalation and exhalation valves are easily damaged by alcohol.

Table 6.5 ACUTE RESPIRATORY HAZARDS

Acetyl chloride	Fluorine	Phosgene
Ammonium hydroxide	Hydriodic acid	Phosphine
Anhydrous ammonia	Hydrobromic acid	Phosphorous chlorides
Arsine	Hydrochloric acid	Phosphorous oxychloride
Bromine	Hydrofluoric acid	
Carbon monoxide	Hydrogen selenide	Sulfur dioxide
Chlorine	Hydrogen sulfide	Sulfur chloride
Chloroform	Hydrogen telluride	Thionyl chloride
	Dimethyl sulfate	Methylfluorosulfonate

6.10.5 ACUTE RESPIRATORY HAZARDS

A number of common substances are acute respiratory hazards and should not be used in a confined area (Table 6.5). These chemicals should be dispensed and handled only with adequate ventilation, in a hood.

6.11 EXAMPLE OF AN EXPOSURE CONTROL PLAN[2,12]

An example of an exposure control plan has been developed in accordance with the OSHA BBP Standard (29 CFR 1910.1030) (Figure 6.4).[2,12]

NOTE: Individuals establishing a BBP program should review the actual standard itself for applicable details for compliance. Information and guidelines for individual laboratory situations must be added where appropriate to establish a complete BBP plan. For obvious reasons, this program example does not include requirements for laboratories engaging in HIV or HBV research and specific instructions for these facilities are to be found within the standard itself.

6.11.1 EXPOSURE DETERMINATION

The exposure determination is made without regard to the use of PPE. (Workers are considered to be exposed even if they wear PPE.) The following job classifications have been identified as those in which workers may be expected to incur exposures, regardless of frequency.

- All physicians
- Laboratory managers and supervisors
- All histology personnel (Figure 6.6)
- Cytology preparation personnel
- All personnel involved in collection, handling, and processing of blood or other potentially infectious materials (Figure 6.7)

Procedures likely to cause exposure to BBPs include:

- Collection, handling, or processing of blood or other potentially infectious materials.
- Autopsy.
- Gross examination of unfixed tissues
- Frozen section procedures
- Cytology specimen preparation

A determination has been made of job classifications for categories "at risk." Personnel must be advised of these categories and are expected to stringently follow practices and procedures that have been assigned to these positions regarding protection from BBPs.

Reviewing the laboratory job descriptions or job classifications, determine which positions represent the different categories of exposure levels:

- I. Routinely experiencing exposure
- II. Experiencing some exposure
- III. Unlikely to experience exposure

Figure 6.4 EXAMPLE OF A BLOODBORNE PATHOGEN PROGRAM EXPOSURE CONTROL PLAN

Facility Name _____

Date of Implementation _____

Authored by _____ Date _____

Authorization by _____ Date _____

Annual Review

Reviewed by _____ Date _____

_____ Date _____

_____ Date _____

_____ Date _____

*(This plan is to be reviewed at least annually and updated as appropriate.)

Figure 6.5 DETERMINING TASK PROTECTIVE REQUIREMENTS

TASK/PROCEDURE	WORK PRACTICE CONTROLS	ENGINEERING CONTROLS	GLOVES LABCOATS	FACE SHIELD	EYE WEAR	OTHER

Figure 6.6 TASK PROTECTIVE REQUIREMENTS: HISTOLOGY LABORATORY

TASK/PROCEDURE	WORK PRACTICE CONTROLS	ENGINEERING CONTROLS	GLOVES LABCOATS	FACE SHIELD	EYE WEAR	OTHER
Accessing Specimens						
Transporting Specimens						
Trimming in Gross Tissue						
Loading Tissue Cassettes						
Disinfecting Gross Area						
Loading Tissue Processor						
Unloading Tissue Processor						
Embedding Tissue						
Sectioning Tissue						
Staining Slides Manual						
Staining Slides Automatic						
Staining-Special						
Staining-Immuno						
Coverslipping Manual						
Coverslipping Automatic						
Handling Covered Slides						
Handling Unfixed Slides						
"Bagging Tissue"						
Disinfecting Work Surfaces/Equipment						
Sectioning Frozen Sections						
Staining Frozen Sections						
Disinfecting Cryostat						
Disinfecting Spills						

Figure 6.7 TASK PROTECTIVE REQUIREMENTS: CLINICAL APPLICATION

TASK/PROCEDURE	WORK PRACTICE CONTROLS	ENGINEERING CONTROLS	GLOVES LABCOATS	FACE SHIELD	EYE WEAR	OTHER
Api Ampulle, opening						
Bone Marrow, assist						
Coulter Operation: Closed Container Open Container						
Container: Transporting Open, ie,Kodak Trays urine tubes Transporting, Closed, ie, Urines, CBCs, Culturettes						
Container: Disposal, Open Disposal, Closed						
Culture: Sputum All othercultures Culture read-out Subbing Cultures						
Diostick UA						
Disinfecting: Work area Daily Instruments Equipment After Spill Biological Waste						
Equipment Maintenance						
Gram Stain						
Monospot, performing						
Pipetting: Body Fluids Chemicals						
Specimens: Aliquoting Racking Recapping						
Smear Preparation						
Stainer: Loading Preparation Cleaning						
Staining, lab						
Throat Screen, performing						
Venipuncture						

Most positions in the laboratory are considered to be those experiencing potential exposure on a routine basis. An exception might be those individuals in administrative or clerical positions who are unlikely to be exposed to the laboratory environment.

Figure 6.8 shows a sample form that can be used to list job descriptions at risk and their levels of exposure.

6.11.2 IMPLEMENTATION SCHEDULE

A schedule of implementation is necessary for compliance with the standard. All controls must be examined and maintained on a regular schedule. [Laboratory Director, Safety Officer, or designated person] will be responsible for examining and maintaining or replacing the engineering control on a/an [weekly, monthly, bimonthly, quarterly, annual] basis to ensure its effectiveness. For example, a schedule of implementation for a BBP exposure plan might be as follows:

- March 6, 1992   Implementation of the plan
- May 5, 1992   Completion of written exposure control plan
- June 4, 1992   Training programs completed and documented
- July 6, 1992   Completion of engineering or work practice changes

6.11.3 ENGINEERING AND WORK PRACTICE CONTROLS

- Controls are utilized to eliminate or minimize exposures to employees in this institution.
- Practices and procedures must be performed in such a manner as to minimize or eliminate splashing, spraying, aerosolization, or production of droplets involving blood or other potentially infectious material.
- No mouth pipetting or suctioning of blood or other potentially infectious material is allowed.
- Handwashing facilities are readily accessible and use is mandatory. Workers must wash their hands immediately or as soon as possible after removal of gloves or other PPE. Workers must wash their hands or other exposed skin surfaces with soap and water or flush mucous

Figure 6.8 DETERMINING JOB CLASSIFICATION FOR CATEGORIES AT RISK

Job Description	Tasks or Procedures	Category of Exposure		
		I	II	III

membranes with water immediately or as soon as possible following an exposure incident.

- Contaminated needles and other contaminated sharps must not be bent, recapped, or removed except in certain circumstances.
- Needles may be recapped using a mechanical device or one-handed technique.
- Needles may be removed using a mechanical device or tool (ie, forceps).
- Contaminated reusable sharps will be placed in appropriate containers immediately after use until decontaminated.
- Workers may not eat, drink, smoke, apply cosmetics or lip balm, or handle contact lenses in the laboratory area.
- Food or drink is not allowed in the laboratory area where blood or other potentially infectious materials may be present.
- Specimens of blood or other potentially infectious material should be placed in leak-proof containers to eliminate potential exposure during collection, handling, or transport. If outside contamination of the primary container occurs, the container must be placed in a secondary container to prevent contamination. (There is an exemption to this labeling/color coding requirement. Because universal precautions require all specimens and containers to be considered potentially infectious, there is no requirement for special labeling. This exemption applies only while specimens remain in the facility.)
- Contaminated equipment (with blood or other potentially infectious material) should be decontaminated before maintenance or servicing.

6.11.4 PERSONAL PROTECTIVE EQUIPMENT

- The following PPE is provided to minimize worker exposure to potentially infectious materials and its appropriate use is mandatory:
  - Disposable gloves
  - Full face masks
  - Head and foot covers
  - Aprons
  - Safety goggles/glasses
  - Laboratory coats
- PPE is provided at no cost to the employee.
- PPE is used based on anticipated exposures.
- PPE must be replaced, repaired, or cleaned as necessary.
- PPE penetrated by blood or other potentially infectious materials must be removed and replaced as soon as possible.
- PPE must be removed before leaving the laboratory area.
- PPE must be placed in designated areas for storage, cleaning, decontamination, or disposal.
- Gloves (latex, vinyl, or hypoallergenic, heavy-duty utility, stainless steel mesh) must be provided and their appropriate use is mandatory.
- Disposable gloves are not to be washed or decontaminated for reuse. Utility and mesh gloves may be decontaminated for reuse if they are examined for damage or defects.
- Gloves are to be replaced as soon as practical when they become contaminated or if they have become barrier compromised.
- Masks in combination with eye protection devices (goggles, full face shields) are required whenever splashes, splatters, or droplets of potentially infectious material are reasonably anticipated.
- Laboratory coats, gowns, and aprons will be used as appropriate.

6.11.5 SIGNS AND LABELING SYSTEMS

- All containers of regulated waste, refrigerators, and freezers used to store, transport, or ship blood or other potentially infectious material must be labeled with the "biohazard" label.
- Red bags or red containers may substitute for labels. (Containers with blood, blood components, or blood products which are labeled as to their contents and released for transfusion or other clinical use are exempt from the labeling requirement.)
- Individual containers of blood or other potentially infectious material that are placed in a labeled container during storage, transport, shipment, or disposal are exempt from individual labeling requirements.
- Contaminated equipment must be labeled and must also state which portion of the equipment remains contaminated.
- Regulated waste that has been decontaminated does not need special labeling.

6.11.6 HOUSEKEEPING AND EQUIPMENT DECONTAMINATION

- Contaminated equipment and work surfaces in each laboratory section must be cleaned and disinfected with [name of product or type of product] after each task or procedure (as appropriate) and at the end of the work shift (Figure 6.9).
- Contaminated instruments and reusable sharps must be cleaned and disinfected with [name of product].
- Receptacles (bins, pails, cans, etc) must be inspected daily and cleaned as soon as possible (feasible) when visibly contaminated.
- Contaminated broken glass must not be picked up with the hands but with mechanical means, such as brush and dust pan, cardboard "pusher" and "receiver," tongs, or forceps.
- Contaminated disposable sharps are discarded in sharps containers.
- Contaminated waste must be placed in appropriate containers as soon as feasible.
- Contaminated laundry must be handled or agitated as little as possible; it is not sorted or rinsed. It is placed in appropriate containers to await removal or pickup. Personnel handling contaminated laundry must wear appropriate PPE.

6.11.7 HBV VACCINATION

- HBV vaccination series is available to all workers who may experience exposure.
- Vaccination is available after worker has been given training and within 10 days of initial work assignment, unless worker has previously had the vaccine or submits to antibody testing that shows the worker to have sufficient immunity.
- Workers may decline the HBV vaccination but may request it at a later date. Workers declining the vaccination must sign a declination statement.

Figure 6.10 shows the steps that must be taken for the administration of the HBV vaccination. Figure 6.11 is a sample form to be filled out at the time of the vaccination.

6.11.8 POSTEXPOSURE EVALUATION AND FOLLOW-UP

If an exposure occurs, it must be reported immediately to the supervisor and safety officer. Exposure incident forms (Figure 6.12) must be prepared and postexposure evaluation must be conducted.

Figure 6.9 DECONTAMINATION SCHEDULE

Section or Unit_____   Verified By_____

EQUIPMENT OR SURFACE	DATE OF DECONTAMINATION	METHOD USED	PERSON RESPONSIBLE	DATE OF NEXT SCHEDULED DECONTAMINATION

6.11.9 EVALUATION BY HEALTH CARE PROFESSIONAL

A written opinion must be obtained from the health care professional who evaluates the worker with regard to obtaining HBV vaccination and whenever a worker is seen following an exposure incident. Health care professionals evaluating workers should be provided with:

- A copy of 29 CFR 1910.1030
- A description of the job as it relates to exposure
- Documentation of the route(s) of exposure and circumstances of the exposure
- Results of the source individual's blood testing, if available
- All medical records relevant to appropriate treatment, including vaccination status

Workers should receive a copy of the health care professional's written opinion within 15 days of completion of the evaluation.

Health care professional's opinion on HBV vaccination should only contain information on whether HBV vaccination is indicated for the worker and if the worker has received the vaccination.

Health care professional's opinion for postexposure evaluation and follow-up indicate only that the worker has been informed of the results of the evaluation and that the worker has been informed of any medical conditions resulting from exposure to blood or other

---

Figure 6.10   STEPS TO BE TAKEN IN THE ADMINISTRATION OF HEPATITIS B VACCINATION[12]

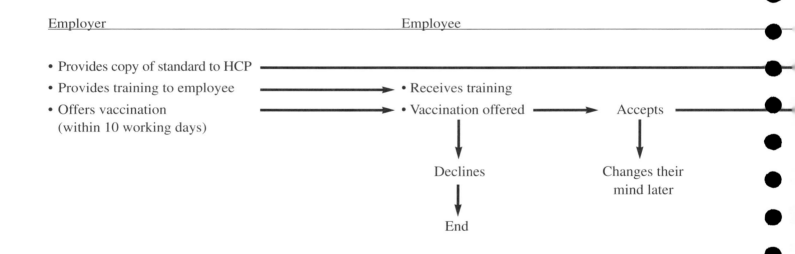

---

potentially infectious materials that require further evaluation or treatment. Any other findings or diagnoses (personal medical information) must remain confidential and must not be included in the written report.

All medical evaluation and procedures, including HBV vaccinations, must be provided to the workers without cost and must be made available at a reasonable time and place under the direction or care of a licensed physician under recommendations of the US Public Health Services.

6.11.10 TRAINING AND EVALUATION

Training for all workers must be provided prior to initial assignment of tasks and at least annually thereafter (Figure 6.13).

Additional training or updates must be provided when there is a change in conditions, procedures, or relevant data regarding exposures.

The training program must include explanation of:
- OSHA BBP Standard
- Epidemiology and symptoms of bloodborne diseases
- Modes of transmission of BBPs
- The BBP plan (exposure control plan) including applicable points of the plan, lines of

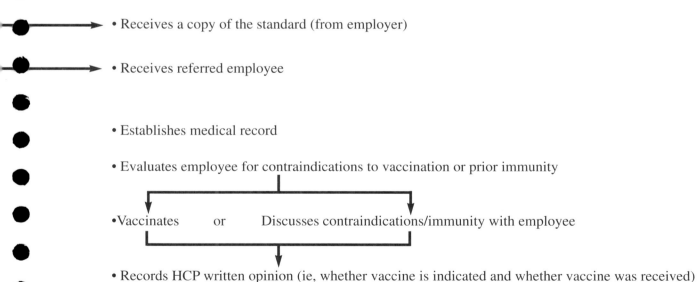

Healthcare Professional (HCP)

- Receives a copy of the standard (from employer)

- Receives referred employee

- Establishes medical record

- Evaluates employee for contraindications to vaccination or prior immunity

- Vaccinates   or   Discusses contraindications/immunity with employee

- Records HCP written opinion (ie, whether vaccine is indicated and whether vaccine was received)
- Provides copy of written opinion to employer

Figure 6.11 EXAMPLE OF A HEPATITIS B VIRUS VACCINATION FORM

Name _____ SS# _____

Address _____

Department _____ Job Title _____

I have received and read the information on hepatitis B and hepatitis B vaccine. I have received instructions and have had the opportunity to ask questions regarding hepatitis B and the hepatitis B vaccine. I understand the benefits, risks, and contraindications for the vaccination. I further understand that I must have three doses of vaccine to confer immunity. However, there is no guarantee that I will become immune or that I will not experience any adverse side effects from the vaccine.

[ ] Yes

I request that the vaccine series be administered to me. (A series of three doses. After the initial dose, the second dose must be administered at 30 days, and the third dose at 180 days from the initial dose.)

[ ] No

I have decided not to receive the vaccination series. I understand that due to my occupational exposure to blood or other potentially infectious materials, I may be at risk of acquiring hepatitis B virus (HBV) infection. I have been given the opportunity to receive the HBV vaccine at no charge to myself. However, I decline vaccination at this time. I understand that by declining this vaccine, I continue to be at risk of acquiring HBV, a serious disease. If, in the future, I continue to have occupational exposure to blood or other infectious materials and I want to be vaccinated with the HBV vaccine, I can receive the vaccination series at no charge to myself.

[ ] I have previously completed the three-dose series of HBV vaccine at another institution.

Name of Facility _____

Address _____

Date of Vaccination _____

Employee Signature _____ Date _____

Witness Signature _____ Date _____

Figure 6.12 SAMPLE POSTINCIDENT EVALUATION AND FOLLOW-UP FORM

Laboratory or Section _____ Date _____

Supervisor _____

Employee _____ SS # _____

Address _____

Date and time of incident _____

Describe circumstances and exposure of the incident _____

_____

What protective equipment was used _____

Route of Exposure _____

[ ] Needlestick, puncture, laceration

[ ] Blood or body fluid contact to skin with breaks, cuts, sores, etc

[ ] Blood or body fluid contact with eyes, nose, or mouth

Source of Exposure _____

[ ] Treated waste (requires first aid only)

[ ] Untreated or unknown status medical waste

[ ] Needlestick, blood or body fluid source

      [ ] Unknown

      [ ] Known

      [ ] Refuses to be tested

      [ ] Consents to testing (HBV, HIV)

      [ ] Test results are negative

      [ ] Test results are positive

Exposure Protocol _____

[ ] First aid: Immediately clean wound and protect

[ ] Exposure incident counseling with employee

Employee is informed of:

      [ ] Potential risk of HIV or HBV infection is very low

      [ ] Test results from source individual (if tested)

      [ ] Results of blood tests and medical evaluation

      [ ] Any medical condition(s) resulting from the incident that would require further evaluation

      [ ] Confidentiality of all phases of follow-up and medical evaluation

      [ ] Need for HIV blood testing and immunization therapy

Figure 6.12 CONTINUED

During follow-up period, employee is advised to:

    [ ] Report to employee any illness that occurs, particularly fever, rash, fatigue, swollen glands, or flu-like symptoms

    [ ] Refrain from donating blood, semen, or body organs

    [ ] Abstain from or use protective measures during sexual intercourse

    [ ] Do not breast feed (if female)

    [ ] Return to employer if any questions or concerns arise

    [ ] Keep all follow-up and scheduled appointments

Follow-up Procedures

HIV precaution

    [ ] Access current status; perform ELISA test

    [ ] If reactive, perform Western blot test to confirm (attach inoculation documentation)

HBV precaution

    [ ] Access current status by vaccination or preexisting immunity

    [ ] Immunity confirmed

    [ ] Confirmation unavailable, test for antibodies to HB surface antigens (anti-HBs)

    [ ] Immunity confirmed

    [ ] Immunity not confirmed, provide HB immune globulin (gluteal intramuscular)

Hepatitis non-A, non-B/hepatitis C (HCV) precaution

    [ ] Give immune globulin

Tetanus precaution

    [ ] Assess current status

    [ ] Booster received within last 5 years, no action

    [ ] Booster received

    [ ] Never received tetanus/diptheria primary series

[ ] Follow-up investigation and evaluation are complete.

[ ] All appropriate testing and inoculations are complete.

[ ] Employee has been informed of all appropriate information.

[ ] All appropriate documentation, testing, and inoculation records are complete.

Verified by   Date

responsibilities, and implementation of the plan
- Procedures that may result in exposures
- Control methods to be used to eliminate or minimize exposure
- PPE available and proper use and maintenance
- Incident reporting procedures and emergency procedures
- Postexposure evaluation and follow-up procedures
- Signs and labels to be used
- HBV vaccination program

6.11.10 A POSTTRAINING TEST

The following is a sample questionnaire that can be administered after training in the BBP Standard has been given. Answers are given at the end of this chapter.

1. The three most common source materials for laboratory acquired HBV or HIV infection are:
   [ ] Blood

Figure 6.13 DOCUMENTATION OF TRAINING IN PROTECTION OF LABORATORY EMPLOYEES FROM BLOODBORNE INFECTIONS[10]

Instructor_____ Department_____

(Name)_____ SS #_____

received training in the protection of laboratory employees from infectious disease transmitted by blood, body fluid, and tissue and has had an opportunity to ask questions from the instructor and understand the principles and goals of the Bloodborne Pathogen Standard.

Date_____ Employee Signature_____

Date_____ Instructor Signature_____

Additional Training Provided

Date_____ Supervisor_____ Employee Signature_____

_____
_____
_____
_____

[ ] Semen

[ ] Tissue

[ ] Urine

[ ] Serum/Plasma

2. HBV infection can usually be prevented by immunization with recombinant hepatitis B vaccine.

[ ] True

[ ] False

3. The most common route of entry of HBV or HIV is by

_____.

4. The risk of HIV infection after a single contaminated needle stick is:

[ ] 6% –30%

[ ] 10%

[ ] 0.4%

[ ] 0.15%

5. HIV survives a relatively short time in dried blood.

[ ] True

[ ] False

6. HBV and HIV can be killed by alcohol, aldehydes, and intermediate-level chlorine germicides.

[ ] True

[ ] False

7. The main feature of universal precautions is

_____ protection.

8. Sharps containers are usually made of _____ plastic, colored _____, and disposed of by _____.

9. AZT is a proven preventive of HIV infection, if given immediately after accidental exposure.

[ ] True

[ ] False

10. Adequate protection for each of the following hazards is provided by the following protective devices. (Match the hazard with the appropriate device[s]).

1. Needle stick	a. Eyeglasses
2. Contamination of hand wound	b. Face mask
3. Airborne transmission of *M tuberculosis*	c. Personal respirator
4. Splashing blood in eyes	d. Latex gloves
5. Soaking-through of blood on clothing	e. Handwashing
	f. Surgical mask
	g. Fluid-resistant lab coat
	h. Heavy-weight utility gloves
	i. None of the above

6.11.11 RECORDKEEPING

All records as required by the OSHA standard are maintained and are the responsibility of [designated person]. (All medical and training records are available to the subject worker.)

6.12 REFERENCES

1. Centers for Disease Control. Guidelines for prevention of transmission of Human immunodeficiency virus and hepatitis B virus to health care and public safety workers. *Lab Med.* November 1989:783-797.
2. Occupational Safety and Health Administration, Department of Labor. *Occupational Exposure to Bloodborne Pathogens: Final Rule.* 20 CFR 1910.1030. Washington, DC. December 1991.
3. Lawson S. Why are OSHA regulations facing such intense scrutiny [revision]? June 1992:19-20.
4. Montgomery L. Bloodborne pathogen standard now in effect. *Histologic.* 1992:332,334.
5. Montgomery L. *The Bloodborne Pathogen Standard: Education and Training Manual.* Jackson, Miss: National Society for Histotechnology; 1993.
6. Fredenburgh J, Grizzle W. *Safety in the Tissue Processing/Histology Laboratory: Toxic Chemicals to Biohazards.* Kalamazoo, Mich: Richard-Allen Industries.
7. National Committee for Clinical Laboratory Standards. *Protection of Laboratory Workers from Infectious Diseases Transmitted by Blood, Body Fluids, and Tissue.* Villanova, Pa: National Committee for Clinical Laboratory Standards; 1991. NCCLS Document M29-T2, Vol 11, No. 14.
8. Montgomery L. Decontamination of potentially infectious spills. *Tech Sample.* 1993;HT-2.
9. Chapman B. Protecting yourself during autopsy. *CAP Today.* July 1993.
10. Tilford M, Bastian F. Handling Cruetzfeldt-Jakob disease tissues in the histology laboratory. *J Histotechnol.* 1989;12:214.
11. Greenblatt M. Questions and Answers. *CAP Today.* March 1993.
12. Occupational Safety and Health Administration, Department of Labor. *Enforcement Procedures for the Occupational Exposure to Bloodborne Pathogens Standard, 20 CFR 1910.1030.* Washington, DC: Occupational Safety and Health Administration; 1992. OSHA Instruction CPL 2-2, 44C.
13. Kuebler D. Decontamination of laboratory equipment. *The Network.* June 1992.
14. Christy E. Outfitted to filter out respiratory risk. *Occup Health Saf.* September 1993.
15. Parker J. Standard for respiratory protection. *Indus Hyg News.* September 1993.
16. Centers for Disease Control. Guidelines for preventing the transmission of tuberculosis in health care settings. *MMWR.* 1990;39(17):1-29.
17. Eisenberg P. Do you make these common mistakes in maintaining your respiratory masks? *Occup Health Saf.* February 1992:43-45.

6.12.1 ADDITIONAL READINGS

Alpert L. AIDS precautions in the 90s: prudence or paranoia? *Med Lab Observer.* May 1992.
Alpert L. Prevention of device-mediated bloodborne infections. *Med Lab Observer.* May 1992:43-45.
Brown J. Compiling employee safety records that will satisfy OSHA. *Med Lab Observer.* June 1992:45-48.
Brown J. Laboratorians: on the front line of exposure. *Med Lab Observer.* August 1991:54-60.
Brown J. Safety protocols no lab can ignore. *Med Lab Observer.* May 1992:27-29.
Brown J. Teaching your staff about biosafety. *Med Lab Observer.* April 1992:24-28.
College of American Pathologists, Environment Safety and Health Committee. *Guidelines for Laboratory Safety.* Skokie, Ill: Subcommittee on Laboratory Resources, College of American Pathologists; 1989.
Hickman S. Innovative ideas for complying with OSHA regs. *Med Lab Observer.* December 1992.
International Society for Clinical Laboratory Technology and the American Association of Bioanalysts. *Guide to OSHA Requirements for Hospital, Independent, and Physician Office Laboratories.* St Louis, Mo: International Society for Clinical Laboratory Technology; 1990.
Kimberly-Clark Corporation. *Mini-Guide to OSHA Final Rule for Occupational Exposures to Bloodborne Pathogens.* Roswell, Ga: Kimberly-Clark Corporation; 1993.

Luebbett PP. When OSHA knocks. *Adv Administrator Labs.* March/April 1993:20-23.

Pugliese G. *OSHA's Final Bloodborne Pathogens Standard: A Special Briefing.* Chicago, Ill: Division of Quality Resources, American Hospital Association; 1992.

Rekus JF. Bloodborne pathogens. *Occup Health Saf.* May 1992:32,34,57.

Rekus JF. Health industry adjusts to specifics of bloodborne pathogen exposure rule. *Occup Health Saf.* June 1992.

Rekus JF. PPE. *Occup Health Saf.* May 1992.

Wallace E. Training: key to reducing risks of occupational exposure to bloodborne pathogens. *Indus Hyg News.* January 1993.

Wilson N, Cavnar P. The economic impact of OSHA's proposed rule on occupational exposure to bloodborne pathogens. *Lab Med.* January 1993;23.

ANSWERS TO 6.11.10 A

1. Blood; tissue; serum/plasma
2. True
3. Needle stick
4. 0.4%
5. False
6. True
7. Barrier protection
8. Rigid/puncture-resistant; red/yellow; incineration
9. False
10. 1. (i) Heavy-weight utility gloves
    2. (d, i) Latex gloves, heavy-weight utility gloves
    3. (c) Personal respirator
    4. (b) Face mask
    5. (h) Plastic surgeons gown

Chapter 7

Procedures for Handling Radiologic Materials

7.1 INTRODUCTION

Radioactive materials are used in therapeutic, diagnostic, and research activities and can include any solid, liquid, or gas emitting radiation. For laboratory purposes, low-level licensed quantities of radioactive material are used. The Nuclear Regulatory Commission (NRC) generally regulates all license activities. However, there are 29 "agreement states" that have approval from the NRC for licensing and enforcing all radioactive materials within their boundaries.[1] The user, therefore, must refer to detailed regulations and instructions from federal and state authorities. The following procedures are suggested as a guideline for the use and handling of radiologic materials in the laboratory.[2] These guidelines are not intended to be all inclusive. The users of radioactive materials must develop their individual detailed safety procedures for use and handling of radiologic materials in accordance with state and federal regulations.[3]

Handling and use of radiologic materials in the anatomic pathology laboratory are limited. It is prudent, however, to be aware of, and have in place, procedures and practices that include the use and handling of radiologic materials if the situation arises. Any radiologic material user should refer to detailed safety procedures such as those available from the NRC.

7.2 WARNING SIGNS AND LABELS

- Warning signs indicating the presence of radioactive materials must be posted in any area storing radionuclides.
- Appropriate labels must be placed on all containers of radionuclide preparations that are made in the laboratory.

7.3 STORAGE AND SECURITY

- Shipments of radioactive material must be received directly by authorized personnel and placed immediately in the isotope storage area.
- Shipments of radionuclides should not be left unattended in any area with access by the public or nonauthorized personnel.
- All shipments of radioactive materials must be placed in approved storage areas or within a lead brick storage area.
- The isotope storage area must be locked whenever authorized laboratory personnel are not in attendance.

7.4 DISPOSAL PROCEDURES

Radiation waste materials are disposed of in compliance with state and federal regulations. The user must consult the radiation safety officer for detailed procedures for proper disposal of these materials. If the facility is not large enough for a radiation office, the laboratory director will act in this capacity. (Consult *Guidelines for Clinical Laboratory Waste Management*; NCCLS Document GP5-A, 1994.)

7.5 HANDLING RADIONUCLIDES

All personnel working with radioactive materials should be registered with the radiation safety office or laboratory director. All personnel must attend radiation safety training before initiation of such work.[2]

7.5.1 LIQUIDS

- Do not pipet or handle directly. Remove liquid from vials with a syringe and needle or automatic pipetting device.
- Leave vials inside lead containers.
- Wash hands immediately after each procedure.

7.5.2 IN VITRO TEST KITS

- The level of radioactivity is generally very low.
- Care must be taken when adding labeled material to test tubes.
- Tubes must be covered with caps.
- *Washing*: Tubes must be flushed with aspirators and washed in drain with adequate amounts of water. Splashing or spraying of any rinse water must be avoided.

7.5.3 CAPSULES

Never handle directly; handle with forceps or plastic/paper cups.

7.5.4 PERSONAL PROTECTIVE EQUIPMENT

- Use laboratory coats or aprons and gloves when handling liquids.
- Change immediately if contamination occurs. Wash or set aside until contamination decays. Check washed coat or aprons with survey meters periodically to detect contamination.

7.6 SPILLS

Capsules are picked up using forceps.

In case of liquids spills:
- Notify the supervisor immediately.
- Evacuate all nonessential personnel.
- Wear gloves and soak up spill with absorbent paper. Place the gloves and absorbent paper in a plastic bag. Place bag behind adequate shielding to decay before disposal.
- Scrub area with soap and water. Rinse thoroughly.
- Survey the area with a rate meter to detect any residual contamination and repeat washing if necessary.
- Wash hands thoroughly. (See also 4.6.1.)

7.7 NOTIFICATION OF POTENTIAL HAZARDS AND PERSONNEL RIGHTS

All personnel handling or exposed to radioactive materials (radionuclides) are notified and instructed regarding the presence and potential hazards of these materials, and all personnel are instructed in the safe handling and use of these materials.

Personnel performing in vitro tests will be required to wear film badges for detection of any contamination.

Personnel will be provided with the following information:
- Reports of exposure records (film badges)
- Reports of any accidental exposure and notice of reports sent to NRC
- They have the right to file complaints regarding these matters.
- They may accompany an NRC inspector during an inspection.

7.7.1 NOTIFICATION AND RESTRICTIONS

Posting of the following notices is required by law:
- Regulations pertaining to notices, instructions, and reports
- License and conditions of use are kept on file in the isotope committee book, the administrator's office, and the laboratory

All notices must be posted on a centrally located bulletin board.

7.7.2 PERSONNEL SAFETY PROCEDURES

- Only those personnel who have been instructed in the proper techniques and safety precautions should handle radioisotopes.
- Persons with open cuts or sores must not handle isotopes unless they are protected or covered by latex gloves.
- No smoking is permitted in the laboratory. This is particularly important in and around the area where radioisotopes are handled.
- Pregnant women are to be advised of the potential reproductive hazard but are not to be excluded from working in the area.

7.8 REFERENCES

1. Furr K, ed. *CRC Handbook of Laboratory Safety.* 3rd ed. Boston, Mass: CRC Press; 1991.
2. Committee for Laboratory Biosafety. *Laboratory Biosafety Guidelines.* Baton Rouge, La: Louisiana State University School of Veterinary Medicine; 1992.
3. Radiation Safety Office. *Campus Radiation Safety Manual.* Baton Rouge, La: Louisiana State University; 1994.

7.8.1 ADDITIONAL READINGS

Nuclear Regulatory Commission. 10 CFR 19. *Notices, Instructions, and Reports to Work Inspections.* January 1, 1994:296-302.

Nuclear Regulatory Commission. 10 CFR 20. *Standards for Protection Against Radiation.* January 1, 1994:302-327.

Nuclear Regulatory Commission. *Prenatal Radiation Exposure.* Regulatory guide No. 8.13.

Department of Transportation. 49 CRF 1-7. *Transportation of Hazardous Waste.* January 1, 1993.

Occupational Safety and Health Administration. 29 CFR 1910.96. *Ionizing Radiation.* July 1, 1993:218-227.

Tuberculosis in the Laboratory

MILLER-MOTTE TECHNICAL
COLLEGE LIBRARY

8.1 OSHA's Compliance Directive

In the past few years, medical laboratory personnel have had to reacquaint themselves with an old enemy that had been considered all but vanished. *Mycobacterium tuberculosis* (TB), until about 1984, had been declining. From 1985 to 1991, the incidence of TB increased by 16%. The aged, poor, and minority populations are disproportionately represented in this group and to a large extent make up current TB patients. Perhaps the greatest contributor to the rise of TB is the continuing increase in the number of human immunodeficiency virus (HIV)–infected persons who make up a large portion of the population in hospitals, prisons, and shelters.[1] *M tuberculosis* outbreaks have led the Centers for Disease Control and Prevention (CDC) to publish new guidelines on preventing transmission in health care settings. Adherence to these guidelines should prevent almost all nosocomial transmission of this organism.[2] These guidelines include significant provisions for respirator use. Protection of "high risk" personnel, which includes most laboratory workers, is assured by providing National Institute for Occupation Safety and Health (NIOSH)/Occupation Safety and Health Administration (OSHA)–approved respirators with high-efficiency particulate air (HEPA) filters.

It is particularly important to know that TB may be present in any unfixed tissue or body fluid specimen received in a laboratory. Any unfixed tissue or body fluid specimens, including lavage, urine, cerebrospinal fluid, and sputum specimens may be potential hazards. Of particular concern are those procedures that require direct handling of unfixed specimens, such as sputum, and frozen section procedures. Aerosols are created when frozen tissue is sectioned. Freezing aerosol products is not appropriate because of further aerosolization within the cryostat chamber. Strict adherence to universal precautions and use of appropriate personal protective equipment (PPE) (NIOSH/OSHA–approved masks, gowns, gloves, and eyewear) is essential. An appropriate biosafety hood should be used when handling any fresh tissue, body fluid, or sputum specimens. Certainly, procedures for personnel engaged in phlebotomy, collection of cytology specimens, fine needle aspiration, and surgical or autopsy procedures must be thoroughly evaluated. Individuals engaged in research must consider the hazards of naturally or experimentally infected nonhuman primate contact as well as those hazards involving cultures of *M tuberculosis* or *M bovis*. Other experimental animals including guinea pigs or mice do not necessarily pose a direct hazard from "coughing" but their contaminated litter may become a source of infectious aerosols to handlers or other personnel.[3]

Whatever laboratory environment is considered, it is important to know the biosafety criteria established for TB. Laboratory biosafety (microbial) criteria have been promulgated by the CDC and are classified into four levels identified as biosafety levels 1 (minimum hazard) through 4 (extreme hazard). Important considerations include:
- *M tuberculosis* (virulent strains) falls into biosafety level 3.
- The drug-resistant strains, which are extremely hazardous for immunosuppressed individuals, and patients with acquired immunodeficiency syndrome (AIDS) and genetic conditions should be considered as level 4 hazards.
- *M tuberculosis*–containing (or suspected) materials are considered to be viable and thus extremely hazardous unless they have been autoclaved, formalinized, treated with a 1:10 solution of hypochlorite (bleach), or lethally incinerated.[4]

Facilities engaged in research activities or high-risk diagnostic services should consult detailed information and instructions regarding the operation and work practices for special biosafety laboratories.

Addressing the recent outbreaks of TB, including a multidrug-resistant strain of the disease, OSHA issued the enforcement policy guidelines for workplace exposure to TB. According to the Department of Labor, five health care workers have died from TB, 16 have developed active multidrug-resistant TB, and at least several hundred workplace-oriented cases of TB have been identified across the country.[5] Initially, OSHA's guidelines were modeled after the 1990 guidelines of the CDC and were effective immediately, with respiratory requirements becoming effective January 18, 1994. A final OSHA compliance directive (based on revised CDC guidelines[6]) was to be issued in January 1994, but was delayed. Following the publication of the "Guidelines for Preventing the Transmission of Tuberculosis in Health Care Facilities, Second Edition,"[7] OSHA issued an enforcement policy,[8] which includes provision for inspections and importantly, the use of the General Duty Clause (Section 5 [a] [1]) and the Personal Protection Regulation to enforce proper respirator use. This enforcement policy of the CDC guidelines serves as the law until the new OSHA Tuberculosis Standard is released in 1995. The new standard is not expected to present any dramatic changes from the present form; however, it will follow the uniform format of other similar standards discussed herein. There may be considerable changes in the information regarding respirators and respirator protection. Readers should be aware of this impending change in the law and obtain a copy of the new standard as soon as it is available so that their compliance programs can be updated. Until that time, however, facilities should follow the CDC guidelines issued in October 1993 for their program compliance.

Larger facilities and hospitals have the advantage of an employee health department and infection control personnel as part of the overall operation of the facility. Obviously, many of these guidelines fall directly under the responsibilities of the employee health and infection control officer, thus relieving the laboratory from developing an entire TB program but instead providing a program to comply and coexist with the facility plan. Smaller laboratories will have to formulate an entire program. In either case, the laboratory should obtain a copy of the guidelines for reference when establishing its programs.

8.2 An Overview of the CDC Guidelines[7]

8.2.1 SCOPE OF THE GUIDELINES

The guidelines cover virtually all types of health care facilities, other facilities and residential settings providing medical care, and all health care workers (paid or unpaid) or students who may be potentially exposed to TB.

8.2.2 DETERMINATION OF RISK ASSESSMENT

This includes the following:
- Development of a TB control plan
- Risk assessment of facility as a whole, sections/areas, and worker groups
- Determination of risk classes (low, intermediate, high risk)
- Case surveillance
- Review of TB patient's medical records

- Review of infection control procedures
- Identification of potentially active TB patients
- Management of ambulatory care, emergency room, and hospitalized patients

8.2.3   ENGINEERING CONTROLS

- Ventilation/air flow from clean to unclean
- Monitor air flow using smoke tubes for air current detection.
- Determine UV or HEPA filtration effectiveness and requirements.

8.2.4   RESPIRATORY PROTECTION PROGRAM

Requirements for equipment include:
- HEPA-filtered masks only, at least three sizes provided
- Individually fit tested with face seal leakage no more than 10%
- One micron size particle filter, efficiency of $\geq 95\%$ with flow rates of up to 50 L per minute

Mask use is required:
- During aerosol-generating procedures
- During surgical (autopsy, etc) procedures on suspect patients
- When engineering controls are not adequate
- During cough-inducing procedures
- In TB isolation rooms
- In emergency vehicle transport

8.2.5   PERSONNEL SCREENING PROGRAM FOR TB

Initial Mantoux Purified Protein Derivative (PPD) two-step booster is required at the time of employment for all employees except workers with documented positive test result, adequate treatment, or adequate preventive treatment.

Negative PPD Test Result:
- Repeat as assigned by risk status determination.
- Inform personnel of test results.

PPD Conversions:
- Test other workers in area or group.
- Repeat every 3 months until negative for two consecutive 3-month periods.

Positive PPD Workers:
- Evaluate for active disease.
- Evaluate for preventive treatment if not active.
- Determine potential point of exposure.
- Evaluate PPD-positive workers periodically.

Personnel with Active Disease:
- Exclude from work while active to return only when clinically inactive.
- Facility is responsible for follow-up with primary care physician.

Personnel with Latent TB:
- May work with active preventive treatment.
- May work if the worker refuses or does not complete treatment, but should be counseled about risk of disease development and reassessed according to risk.

8.2.6 POSTEXPOSURE PROCEDURES

- Assess personnel for potential facility transmission
- Provide PPD to workers and/or patients exposed
- If previously PPD-positive, no need to retest, follow up clinically
- Investigate and identify source of exposure and methods to prevent future exposures

8.2.7 TRAINING AND EDUCATION REQUIREMENTS

- Basic knowledge of TB
- Significance of preventive treatment and drug treatment for TB. Table 8.1 lists some commonly used methods to prevent transmission of TB in the laboratory
- Potential for occupational exposures, the immunocompromised worker, anergy in immune function decline
- Infection control procedures and TB plan
- PPD testing program
- Responsibility of ill or PPD-positive personnel
- Policy for voluntary duty reassignment for immunocompromised personnel such as HIV-positive workers
- Confidentiality

Table 8.1 METHODS TO PREVENT TRANSMISSION OF TUBERCULOSIS IN THE LABORATORY[2]

Treat all specimens as potentially infectious, particularly respiratory tract specimens.

Use a biological safety cabinet for processing and handling specimens.

Use safety cups during centrifugation.

Wear gloves when handling all specimens, particularly respiratory tract specimens.

Wear laboratory coats that are tight at the wrist with gloves covering the cuff.

Wear appropriate face shields, safety goggles, and masks.

Do not wear work shoes in your home.

Always wash hands after removing gloves.

Do not sniff sputum specimens or cultures grown from the respiratory tract.

Do not work in an area that lacks appropriate work space.

Decontaminate work surfaces and equipment frequently.

Decontaminate sputum or body fluid spills immediately.

Evacuate the area immediately if specimens are dropped outside the biological cabinet.

8.3   OSHA Enforcement Policies[8]

OSHA will inspect for TB infection hazard controls during compliance inspections as well as investigate employee complaints. Prompted by increasing private sector and health care facility concerns, these new guidelines include replacing the use of standard surgical masks with particulate respirators in health care facilities.[1] State enforcement agencies must advise OSHA of how they will enforce TB infection controls by November 1993. Compliance officers must apply OSHA warning and recordkeeping standards for TB inspections and also follow the General Duty Clause, which obligates employers to free facilities of known hazards.

Controls will mandate protocols for the following:
- Identification of suspected TB cases with symptoms listed by the CDC
- Employee training and education in TB transmission and control
- Initiation of Mantoux skin tests
- Work restrictions and practices for infectious employees
- Negative-pressure respiratory isolation rooms for suspected or confirmed infectious TB patients
- Use of HEPA respirators and respirator training (29 CFR 1910.134)

All laboratories should obtain a copy of the enforcement policy guidance on workplace exposure to TB. Copies can be obtained from OSHA Publications Office (202) 219-5655.

8.4   Methods of Compliance[4]

8.4.1   ESSENTIAL SAFETY PRACTICES

- All known or suspected *M tuberculosis*–containing specimens are to be handled in isolation using special precautions.
- All procedures or manipulation of known or suspected *M tuberculosis*–containing specimens are to be conducted in a biological safety cabinet or other physical containment device. No work is allowed on open bench surfaces. Biological safety cabinets are to be used (1) during procedures with a potential for creating infectious aerosols (grinding, blending, vigorous shaking or mixing, sonic disruption, and opening of containers with potentially infectious materials) and (2) whenever large volumes or high concentrations of potentially infectious materials are handled.
- All personnel working with suspected or known *M tuberculosis* specimens are required to wear PPE such as laboratory coats, masks, safety glasses, gloves, and respirators if appropriate. PPE must be removed before leaving the laboratory area.
- Laboratory access is limited to authorized personnel only.
- Special care must be taken to avoid skin contamination from potentially infectious materials. Gloves are always worn when working with these specimens.
- Gloves are to discarded into biohazard containers. Gloves are not to be used when answering telephones, opening doors, or handling other noncontaminated items.
- Needles must not be bent, shared, replaced in the sheath or guard, or removed from the syringe following use. Needles and syringes will be placed immediately after use in puncture-resistant containers and decontaminated (preferably autoclaved) before disposal.

- Appropriate biohazard containers are to be used.
- Only mechanical pipetting devices are to be used.
- Every effort is to be made to minimize or prevent aerosolization of potentially infectious materials.
- All work surfaces should be decontaminated immediately after use with an appropriate decontaminate such as 1:10 bleach solution.

8.4.2 CENTRIFUGATION PROCEDURES

Materials may be centrifuged in the open laboratory when safety cups or appropriately sealed tubes are used. Tubes are opened only in a biological safety cabinet.

8.4.3 POTENTIALLY INFECTIOUS BIOMEDICAL SPILL PROCEDURES

- Notify supervisor and safety officer immediately.
- Clean areas of bodies of personnel exposed to spill with a germicidal soap. Refer employee to a health care professional for evaluation if appropriate.
- Trained personnel with appropriate PPE (coats, gloves, masks, boots, and respirator if appropriate) should clean the area.
- Thoroughly disinfect the area with a 1:10 bleach solution.

8.4.4 POTENTIALLY INFECTIOUS WASTE

- Potentially infectious liquid waste may be disposed of into sewage system after decontamination by autoclaving. (Get written permission from local sewage system operator.) Tissues that are potentially infectious must be incinerated. (Any generator operating its own incinerator must be licensed by the state health officer.) All bags and other containers of potentially infectious biomedical waste (PIBW) must be labeled "Potentially Infectious Waste" or "Infectious Waste."
- Untreated PIBW that leaves the premises of the generator must be labeled with the name and address of the generator. Treated, but still recognizable, PIBW must carry a supplemental label to specify the treatment method used and name of the person responsible for treatment.
- PIBW must be stored in a secure manner and location.
- A contingency plan must be implemented for periods of 1 day, 7 days, 29 days, and more than 30 days if incineration or other means of on-site destruction are inoperative for any reason.
- Treatment by steam sterilization should include autoclaving at a temperature of at least 120°C at a pressure of at least 15 psi for at least 30 minutes. Treatment by chemical disinfection must be with written permission of the state health officer. The exception is disinfection using a 1:10 bleach solution. Permission must be obtained from the operating authority of the local sewage system for drain disposal.
- Treatment of sharps is by incineration.
- Treated PIBW may be disposed of as nonhazardous waste in a permitted sanitary landfill in accordance with Environmental Protection Agency requirements.

8.5 REFERENCES

1. Brown J, Body B. Tuberculosis alert: an old killer returns. *Med Lab Observer.* May 1993:53-60.
2. McCombs W. Tuberculosis: an increasing health risk. *Scott and White Lab Q.* 1993;5(1):1-2,11.
3. Chapman C. Tuberculosis update. *Mass Soc Histotechnol Newsletter.* 1994;18(4) .
4. Committee for Laboratory Biosafety. *Laboratory Biosafety Guidelines.* Baton Rouge, La: Louisiana State University School of Veterinary Medicine; 1992.
5. Tuberculosis speeds enforcement. *Occup Health Saf.* December 1993.
6. US Department of Health and Human Services. *Recommended Guidelines for Personal Respiratory Protection of Workers in Health Care Facilities Potentially Exposed to Tuberculosis, Centers for Disease Control.* Atlanta, Ga: National Institute for Occupational Safety and Health; 1992.
7. Centers for Disease Control and Prevention. Guidelines for preventing the transmission of tuberculosis in health care facilities, second edition. *Federal Register.* 1993; 58(195):52810-52854.
8. Occupational Safety and Health Administration. *OSHA Enforcement Policy.* Washington, DC: Department of Labor; 1993.

8.5.1   ADDITIONAL READINGS

Centers for Disease Control and Prevention. National action plan to combat multidrug-resistant tuberculosis. *MMWR.* 1992;41 (RR-11):1.

Centers for Disease Control and Prevention. *TB Facts for Healthcare Workers.* Atlanta, Ga: National Center for Disease Prevention Services, Division of Tuberculosis Elimination; 1993.

Centers for Disease Control and Prevention. *NIOSH Recommended Guidelines for Personal Respiratory Protection of Workers in Health Care Facilities Potentially Exposed to Tuberculosis.* Atlanta, Ga: National Institute for Occupational Safety and Health; 1992:1-55.

National Institute for Occupational Safety and Health. *Guidelines for Preventing the Transmission of Tuberculosis in Health Care Settings, With Special Focus on HIV- Related Issues.* Atlanta, Ga: NIOSH; 1990.

Tompkins N. Tuberculosis' comeback alarms public health care professionals. *Occup Health Saf.* March 1993:115,116,133.

Chapter 9

Latex Sensitivity

9.1 ETIOLOGY OF LATEX SENSITIVITIES

Laboratory personnel have experienced a dramatic increase in the incidence of latex-associated dermatitis. These conditions are of concern among laboratory professionals for whom extensive glove use is an occupational necessity. Laboratories must carefully examine their procedures and protocols for glove use and determine those activities in which glove use may be eliminated or modified, or alternative methods or products used.

The National Institute of Occupational Safety and Health has estimated that between 1,070,000 and 1,650,000 injuries to the skin occur annually in the workplace (1988).[1] Skin diseases reduce work efficiency, result in increased absenteeism, often result in downgrading to less skilled positions, and may cause permanent incapacity. Skin diseases account for almost 40% of all reported occupational illnesses in the United States, at an annual cost of more than $1 billion in lost productivity, medical care, and disability payments.[2] Hand dermatitis is the most common occupational skin disease among medical personnel.

Occupation-induced skin disease is not a new phenomenon in the workplace. Actor Buddy Ebsen was unable to play the part of the "Tin man" in the *Wizard of Oz* because he had an allergic skin reaction to the aluminum-based makeup that was necessary for the costume. Allergic reactions are triggered when allergy sufferers come into contact with a substance (or substances) to which they are allergic. When individuals are exposed to an allergen, their bodies will produce histamine in an effort to rid the body of the allergen. Histamine is the substance responsible for creating the symptoms of an allergic reaction.[1] The acquired immunodeficiency syndrome (AIDS) epidemic has led to a dramatic increase in the use of latex rubber gloves and this increased use may be responsible for the rise in the number of cases of allergic contact dermatitis.

In the United States, 8 to 10 billion latex rubber gloves were used in 1988. Latex gloves are preferred over vinyl or plastic gloves because workers believe they fit better, are more durable, and provide a better sense of "touch." However, evidence indicates that there is a substantially higher risk of developing allergic contact dermatitis from the use of latex gloves than from plastic gloves.[1] In addition, the Food and Drug Administration (FDA) has indicated that it will no longer permit the use of terms such as "hypoallergic" on medical devices containing latex, including gloves. This terminology may be misleading with respect to testing claims made by manufacturers that are not an appropriate measure of latex sensitivity.

To investigate incidences of latex allergies, the FDA issued a medical alert on latex gloves advising health care professionals to identify their latex-sensitive patients and be prepared to treat allergic reactions promptly.[3]

The International Latex Conference on Sensitivity to Latex in Medical Devices (November 5-7, 1992, Baltimore, Maryland) was held to obtain knowledge on allergic reactions to latex medical devices. The conference was sponsored by the FDA and cosponsored by the Centers for Disease Control and Prevention (CDC) and National Institute of Allergy and Infectious Disease. Concern was expressed over the increasing evidence of anaphylaxis associated with radiologic procedures, anesthesia, and operative procedures, and sensitization of some health care workers. The combined efforts of medical professionals to identify the problems of latex allergies have produced valuable information.

- Health care workers are one of the main risk groups of latex allergy. Sensitization may occur from the use of protective latex gloves; atopic workers especially and those with hand dermatitis are at risk of developing latex allergy.[4]
- Sensitivities were identified in children with spina bifida, probably as a result of exposure to latex devices early in the treatment of their disorder.
- Gradual sensitization is now being identified in the health care worker. (1% of the general population and 5% to 10% of the health care workers are latex-sensitive.)
- Sensitivity among health care workers may be increasing because of growing use of latex gloves to reduce the risk of AIDS transmission.

9.2 HYPERSENSITIVITY REACTIONS TO LATEX

Type IV: Delayed hypersensitivity, a hapten reaction to chemical additives, can be a risk factor for the more severe type I reaction.

Type I: Hypersensitivity reactions include severe anaphylactic response and are IgE mediated.

9.2.1 "WHY NOW" AFTER YEARS OF USE?

Latex products contain some, but not all, of the nonrubber materials originally present in the concentrate, and also contain some chemicals added to aid processing and affect vulcanization. Interactions may occur between the added chemicals and the proteins. Some of the additives, particularly vulcanization accelerators, can themselves cause allergic reactions in a small proportion of people (usually type IV reactions). The amount of extractable protein remaining in a dipped latex product (gloves, condoms) is highly variable due to differences in manufacturing processes. Manufacturers are currently attempting to modify their processes in order to minimize proteins in their products, which may help prevent sensitization of persons in the future but will not solve the problems of existing sensitized individuals.[2,4] There is a strong correlation between the publication of the CDC's universal precaution recommendations (1987) and proliferation of latex sensitization among health care workers.[4] Several studies indicate risk factors of medication allergies (sulfa, cephalosporins), environmental allergies and food allergies (fruits), atopic reactions, and previous history of contact dermatitis in developing type I allergic reactions.

9.2.2 SYMPTOMS ASSOCIATED WITH REACTIONS TO LATEX GLOVES

- Classic contact dermatitis (eczematic or keratotic form typically crests about 48 hours after contact)
- Contact urticaria syndrome (broad spectrum of reactions, such as wheel/flare reaction within 30 to 60 minutes, dyshidrotic vesiculation, erythema, and itching/burning within 10 to 30 minutes of contact)
- Systemic reactions (nonlocal reactions including generalized urticaria or pruritus, rhinoconjunctivitis, asthma, chest tightness as well as anaphylaxis, eg, hypotension, shock, respiratory failure)

9.2.3 IMMUNOLOGIC ETIOLOGY OF LATEX SENSITIVITY

- Contact dermatitis reactions are T-cell mediated, delayed hypersensitivity reactions.
- Systemic reactions appear to be classic allergic antibody (IgE) mediated.

9.2.4   OTHER SOURCES OF REACTIONS

Powders from latex gloves may be a hidden source of latex protein that can initiate an allergic reaction while some chemicals used in the production of latex products are capable of causing significant reactions themselves.

Dry lubricants (corn starch), sterilizing chemicals (ethylene oxide), and endotoxins found in rubber and curing process chemicals such as accelerators and antioxidants have all been reported as etiologic agents for both local and systemic reactions.

9.3   DIAGNOSTIC PROBLEMS ASSOCIATED WITH LATEX ALLERGY

Symptoms are variable and often mild, causing delay in diagnosis. Health care workers with undiagnosed latex allergic reactions seem not to be at risk to develop severe systemic reactions in their routine work but the risk of intraoperative anaphylaxis is apparent among this group.[4]

9.4   METHODS FOR PREVENTION OR MINIMIZATION OF ALLERGIC REACTIONS TO LATEX

- Prevent persons from becoming latex allergic by (a) reducing or eliminating latex allergen exposure with improved manufacturing processes or development of substitute products; (b) providing nonlatex gloves (vinyl, synthetic, neoprene, etc); (c) maintaining a list of latex-containing products in the workplace and providing alternatives if possible. "Hypoallergic" gloves may not prevent latex reactions. (Labeling claims must be FDA approved and even this is under re-evaluation because of reports of allergic reactions in latex-sensitive individuals.)
- Symptomatic patients should practice latex avoidance and should wear medical identification indicating latex allergy.
- Equipment sources free of latex should be developed for these patients.
- Medical and consumer products containing latex should be labeled.
- Appropriate intervention should be planned for latex-sensitive workers to modify work environment to reduce or eliminate latex exposure.
- If latex gloves must be used, wear vinyl gloves next to skin, then the latex gloves. Cloth liners may also be used.
- Use certain hand creams that have been developed to prevent irritation.
- Switching brands of latex gloves may prove helpful for some individuals.
- Determine if perceived benefit of latex glove use justifies continuing unnecessary exposure to latex through examination gloves.
- The CDC and FDA continue to collect data on latex allergy. To report allergic reactions to latex gloves, call the FDA Product Reporting Program through the US Pharmacopeia at (800) 638-6725.
- Laboratory personnel must be informed of the potential dangers associated with the use of latex gloves in the workplace. They should be informed not only of the possible allergic dermatitis that may develop but also of the very serious allergic reactions reported in some individuals. (See also 5.6.5.)

NOTE: Allergic dermatitis is an important health hazard to health care workers; however, a less discussed, but related, health hazard may be the effect of medical treatment of the allergic reaction itself. Antihistamines used to treat the reactions are available from both the physician and over the counter. While these medications may provide relief from the allergic reaction—sneezing; itching sensations in the nose, throat, and eyes; and watery eyes—they may also result in drowsiness, sedation, blurred vision, and functional impairment. These symptoms primarily result from the use of over-the-counter drugs; nonsedating antihistamines are available from a physician. Individuals receiving treatment for allergic reactions must consider the hazards of working in the laboratory under the influence of any medication that may impair their performance or judgment.

9.5 REFERENCES

1. ECRI. *Dermatitis from Medical Gloves Causes Rash of Worker Complaints.* Plymouth Meeting, Pa: ECRI Publications; 1991.
2. McCallister R. Skin exposures can develop into dermatitis. *Occup Health Saf.* April 1993:71-73.
3. Center for Devices and Radiological Health (HFZ-30), Food and Drug Administration (FDA). Medical alert issued on allergic reactions to latex-containing medical devices. *Med Devices Bull.* April 1991;3:1-2.
4. Culver J. International Latex Conference: sensitivity to latex in medical devices. *J Occup Hosp Health.* 1993;13(1).

9.5.1 ADDITIONAL READINGS

Adams R. Hand eczema: the atopic subject and work. *Cutis.* 1993;52:267-269.

Berky ZT, Luciano WJ, James WD. Latex glove allergy. *JAMA.* 1992;268.

Boxer M. The dangers of latex allergy. *Emerg Med Clin North Am.* July 1993:18-26.

Bubak ME. Allergic reactions to latex among healthcare workers. *Mayo Clin Proc.* 1992;61:1075-1079.

Fisher A. A "Current Contact News" follow-up: controversial subjects and those resulting in litigation. *Cutis.* 1993;52:254-256.

Gonzalez E. Latex hypersensitivity: a new and unexpected problem. *Hosp Pract [Off].* February 1992.

Hamann C, Kick S. Update: immediate and delayed hypersensitivity to natural rubber latex. *Cutis.* 1993;52:307-311.

Larson E. Reported cases of allergic reactions to latex gloves on the rise. *Infect Control Hosp Epidemiol.* August 1991.

Shama SK. Hand dermatitis from gloves. *Occup Environ Med Rep.* May 1991:45-48.

Slater J. Rubber anaphylaxis. *N Engl J Med.* 1989;320:1126-1130.

Slater J. Allergic reactions to natural rubber. *Ann Allergy.* 1992;68:203.

Slater J. Latex allergy: what do we do? *J Allergy Clin Immunol.* 1992;90.

Storrs F. All the things I know were true about contact dermatitis that aren't. *Cutis.* 1993;52:301-305.

Sussman GL, Tarlo S, Dolovich J. The spectrum of IgE-mediated responses to latex. *JAMA.* 1991;265:2844.

Swanson MC, Bubak ME, Hurt LW, Reed CE. Occupational respiratory allergic disease from latex. *J Allergy Clin Immunol.* 1992;89.

Turjanmaa K. Allergens in latex surgical gloves and glove powder. *Lancet.* 1990;336:1588.

Turjanmaa K. Incidence of immediate allergy to latex gloves in hospital personnel. *Contact Dermatitis.* 1987;17:270-275.

Wheeler K. Barrier lotions, along with gloves, can help deter occupational dermatitis. *Occup Health Saf.* January 1992:60-61.

Chapter 10

Waste Minimization and Management

10.1 INTRODUCTION TO WASTE MANAGEMENT

In light of legislative and regulatory agency mandates that have been placed on laboratory operations in the past few years, minimization and management of waste products generated by laboratories have become significant factors determining the overall operations of the laboratory. Included herein is information regarding these issues with an emphasis on areas that may have an impact on the anatomic pathology laboratory. In the interest of brevity, guidelines for radioactive materials have been mentioned but not discussed in great detail in this text. Few anatomic pathology laboratories have significant need for these guidelines and because of the highly technical nature of the subject, it is recommended that laboratories consult detailed guidelines on the matter.

The laboratory is one of the principal generators of hazardous waste (HW) and nonhazardous waste (NHW) in health care facilities. In solid waste alone, a laboratory generates an average of 51.7 lb per day with larger facilities producing up to 1400 lb per day, equaling 30,000 tons of solid waste per year. The Environmental Protection Agency (EPA) estimates that 70% of the landfills existing in 1993 will close within 15 years and that at least 27 states will run out of any landfill facility within 5 years.[1] This presents the laboratory with a very serious mandate to develop methods to minimize, eliminate, and otherwise manage laboratory waste effectively. It is the responsibility of each health care worker to be aware of these problems and conscientiously strive to develop or enhance already existing waste management systems.

Much of the information included in this section is found in *Clinical Laboratory Waste Management: Approved Guidelines,* published by the National Committee for Clinical Laboratory Standards (NCCLS).[1] It is strongly recommended that each laboratory obtain a copy of this document for details regarding specific topics or questions. Table 10.1 lists some of the major federal regulations that have an impact on waste disposal.

10.1.1 CONSIDERATION OF LIABILITY

A discussion of waste minimization and management must address the seriousness of potential liability when disposing of any laboratory waste. Several points must be thoroughly understood when considering disposal problems. These include the following:
- Once waste has been generated (or produced) it is the responsibility of the generator (laboratory) to store, treat, or dispose of waste according to EPA regulations.
- The responsibility remains forever with the generator (laboratory) of the waste.
- The liability may never be transferred (ie, waste hauler). It may become "shared" liability if the waste hauler performs illegally but still the laboratory is responsible.
- Personnel disposing of waste illegally may be personally liable and managers who are aware of illegal practices and do nothing about it are subject to civil and criminal prosecution.

10.1.2 WHO IS A WASTE GENERATOR?

With regard to regulatory agencies, it is first necessary to determine who is a waste generator. Two definitions of waste generator must be considered:
- *Small Waste Generator*: A facility that produces 100 kg but less than 1000 kg of waste per month. A facility that generates over 1000 kg of waste per month is considered a large waste generator.

Table 10.1   Federal Waste Disposal Regulations*

Name of Act	Year	Description
Clean Air Act	1990	Requires EPA to develop rules for emissions from laboratories.
Clean Water Act	1988	Mandated to restore and maintain the physical, chemical and biological integrity of the nation's waters and control nonpoint source of emissions.
Solid Waste Disposal Act	1965	
Resource Recovery Act	1970	
Resource Conservation and Recovery Act (RCRA)	1976	Provides for EPA's authority for HW control.
Hazardous Solid Waste Amendments (HSWA)	1984	
Subtitle C		Regulates hazardous chemical waste.
Subtitle D		Regulates recognized solid waste landfills.
Subtitle J		Regulates medical waste (only 5 states).
Comprehensive Environmental Response, Compensation and Liability Act (CERCLA)(Superfund)		Authorizes EPA to clean up HW spills and inactive (abandoned) HW sites.
Superfund Amendments and Reauthorization Act (SARA)	1986	Establishes community right-to-know of industrial hazards in neighborhoods.
Hazardous Waste Transportation Act	1975	Regulates transportation of hazardous materials in commerce.

Other Federal Laws/Agencies that Affect Hazardous Waste Disposal

NRC	
OSHA Bloodborne Pathogen Standard	
Medical Waste Tracking Act	Defines and regulates medical waste.
Toxic Substance Control Act (TSCA) 1976	Requires public notice of hazard assessment or development of new chemicals
Code of Federal Regulations (CFR)†	Consolidates previously described laws as they apply to laboratories into the CFR
EPA Hazardous	Regulates Medical Waste Tracking (Title 40 [259]) and
	Waste Management Systems
NRC	Title 10 (19, 20)
DOT	Title 49 (171-179): Transportation
OSHA	Title 29 (1910.141): General Waste Disposal
	Title 29 (1910.132): Personal Protective Equipment
	Title 29 (1910.145): Specification of Accident Prevention
	Title 29 (S1200): Hazard Communication
	Title 29 (1910.1030): Bloodborne Pathogen Standard
	Title 29 (1910.1450): Hazardous Substances in Laboratories

Table 10.1 (CONTINUED)

STATE VS FEDERAL REGULATIONS

States are authorized, at least partly, to administer EPA regulations.

Many states have their own plans.

Radionuclides are regulated by some states (with NRC approval).

Incinerators most commonly are regulated by states (EPA may apply).

LOCAL REGULATIONS

Sanitary Sewer Codes	Any laboratory discharging hazardous waste must check with and comply with local codes.
Fire Codes	Usually use regulations established by the NFPA.
NFPA Code 30	Regulates flammable use and storage in laboratories.
Transportation of HW	Special restrictions may prevail at the local level.
Incinerator Emissions	Local laws may be more stringent than those under the Clean Air Act.
Sanitary Landfills	Restrictions usually are on the operator with local jurisdiction over its operation.

EPA = Environmental Protection Agency; HW = Hazardous Waste; NRC = Nuclear Regulatory Commission
OSHA = Occupational Safety and Health Administration; NFPA = National Fire Protection Agency
† For copies of these documents call Government Printing Office (202) 783-3238.

- *Medical Waste Generator*: Under the Medical Waste Tracking Act (1988), a waste generator is defined by occupation rather than by quantity. This is defined as health care provider, veterinarian, research laboratory, or facility involved in treating, diagnosing, or immunizing humans or animals in a participating state.

10.1.3 A SUITABLE TRANSPORTER, TREATMENT, AND DISPOSAL FACILITY[1]

Selecting an appropriate transporter, treatment, and disposal facility is very serious business. Take the time to completely investigate and examine the services provided, the legal regulatory mandates and the overall operation of each service considered. Never settle on a company without receiving at least three bids from other companies for comparison. Remember, the waste generator (the laboratory) is forever responsible for the appropriate disposal of its waste! Qualifications for a suitable service should include:

- Licensing by the state and EPA (mandatory)
- Number of years in business and fiscal stability
- Number and nature of violations cited
- Appropriate recordkeeping, forms, security, manifests, charges, etc
- References from other clients

- Liability insurance
- Initial and on-going training and education provided workers
- Services provided and costs of these services
- Frequency of pickups, emergency pickup availability

10.1.4 DEVELOPING A WASTE MANAGEMENT PROGRAM

- Categories of waste must be defined: Chemical, infectious, radioactive, sharps, or nonhazardous waste.
- For each category of HW define the following: characteristics of the waste; handling (ie, engineering controls, packaging and labels, containment, and personal protective equipment [PPE]); accumulation at point of use; treatment on- and off-site; storage; transportation; disposal; waste minimization and hazard abatement; contingency plans; and regulations and exemptions as appropriate.
- Universal precautions must be adapted to meet local/state regulations.
- Workers must have an understanding of the specific guidelines mandated.

10.1.4 A RESPONSIBILITIES OF THE EMPLOYER

- The employer must develop, establish, and implement a management system to collect, segregate, store, transport, dispose of, and monitor laboratory waste, provide quality assurance, and maintain records.
- The employer must define smaller quantities and use of nonhazardous materials.

10.1.4 B RESPONSIBILITIES OF THE EMPLOYEE

- To comply with procedures
- To segregate, pack, label all waste
- To notify unsafe conditions to managers
- To identify opportunities for HW reduction

10.2 WASTE MANAGEMENT SYSTEMS

The laboratory must develop and implement a system by which HW and NHW is eliminated, minimized, neutralized, or recycled. The plan will not only benefit the health and safety of health care workers and the general public, but will also meet environmental requirements and result in a positive economic impact on laboratory operations.

The purpose of a waste management system is to provide a comprehensive program that addresses environmental concerns and demonstrates the desirability of recycling. The first step in developing a program for waste management is to perform a survey of all waste materials generated by the laboratory, review the processes and procedures that produce waste (hazardous or not), determine what hazardous substances are being used (type and amount), determine what methods are being used for the handling, segregation, storage, on-site treatment and disposal, transfer, and transportation of these wastes (Figure 10.1).[1]

One of the most prominent areas of waste management in the anatomic pathology laboratory is the use of chemical reagents, particularly solvents. In recent years, dramatic advances have been made in the recycling technology available to laboratories. Fractional distillation of solvents such as xylene, xylene substitutes, and alcohols has been demonstrated to provide an exceptional method for not only reducing the HW generated but more importantly, has significantly reduced the overall cost of chemical reagent use through the reclamation of pure solvents and practically eliminated the cost of disposal service removal. Advances in recycling or reclaiming formalin have shown remarkable promise. The availability of formalin substitutes and xylene substitutes has changed the face of laboratory inventories forever. A number of very suitable substitutes have been developed but it must be understood that these products are not without their own hazardous properties and disposal problems. For these products to perform the function intended, the very chemical nature of these reagents cannot be produced without some hazardous effects such as skin, eye, or respiratory problems.

Disposal of these reagents requires careful consideration. The material safety data sheets (MSDSs) must be carefully evaluated and the local water board or municipality must be contacted regarding disposal in sewer systems. Reagents dumped into these systems must not inhibit bacterial growth in biological treatment facilities. They must also have a low or nonexistent aquatic toxicity and be biodegradable in a reasonable period of time. (Beware of products that claim drain disposal if they do not appear on EPA lists of hazardous chemicals. That may mean that it simply hasn't been tested yet!) Carefully evaluate any new products and product claims before introducing any substitute into laboratory operation. However, those substitutes that do provide an appropriate alternative to xylene and formalin, although

---

Figure 10.1   SAMPLE SURVEY FORM FOR WASTE MANAGEMENT SYSTEM

Date _____   Laboratory Section _____

Verified by _____

[ ] Chemical Waste

[ ] Infectious Waste

[ ] Nonhazardous Waste   [ ] Other Considerations _____

[ ] Sharps   _____

[ ] Radioactive Waste   _____

Waste Product	Amt/Wk	Amt/Mo	Method of Treatment	Disposal Method

more expensive, may provide considerable benefits because of the increased costs of compliance (medical hazards, monitoring, and labeling requirements).

The following guidelines outline the steps that must be taken when establishing a waste management program for a laboratory.

10.2.1 DEVELOP THE WASTE MANAGEMENT PROGRAM[1,2]

- Describe the scope, goals, and objectives of the program.
- Meet requirements of the Joint Commission for the Accreditation of Healthcare Organizations and the College of American Pathologists.
- Define a plan to minimize waste hazards and encourage recycling.

10.2.2 INITIAL CONSIDERATIONS

- *Regulatory compliance*, which includes the following:
  - Plan must be developed by knowledgeable person(s).
  - Most cost-effective alternatives that can be used must be incorporated.
  - Must interact with other overlapping/existing/or future programs.
- *Development and implementation*, including:
  - Reviews and approval by all represented departments and managers.
  - Phased approach usually best.
  - Obtain equipment and supplies.
  - Contact outside services such as disposal services.
  - Training and education program.
  - Update and review as appropriate.

10.2.3 DEFINE PROGRAM SPECIFICS[1]

Table 10.2 lists the specific steps that must be included in a waste program.

The rules and regulations for managing hazardous waste are complex, but there is help readily available. For more information, call:
- The state hazardous waste management agency
- The regional EPA office
- The Resource Conservation and Recovery Act (RCRA)/Superfund hot-line ([800] 424-9346)
- EPA's Small Business Ombudsman hot-line ([800] 368-5888)
- The national trade association or its local chapter

10.3 TRAINING AND EDUCATION IN WASTE MANAGEMENT

Essential contents of any waste management plan should include regulatory requirements and accreditation standards, consider liabilities and risks, address the financial demands on the laboratory, and develop a plan that is acceptable to both the personnel and the general public. Training and education of personnel should reflect these objectives. Constantly changing regulations and expanding technologies increase the demands on this process, making training and educational programs a vital part of an on-going program.[1]

Table 10.2 WASTE PROGRAM SPECIFICS

REDUCE USAGE

Elimination, substitution, or reduction of amounts used

Redistillation of solvents and fixatives

Disposal of outdated chemicals

SEGREGATION

Hazardous from nonhazardous waste

Collection of recyclable products

Sharps in containers for sharps only

HANDLING

Safe work practices

Personal protective equipment

Training and education

STORAGE

Reduced number of disposal service pickups

Secure storage areas

TRANSPORTATION

Only authorized disposal service

Manifests, files maintained for 3 years

Generators of waste forever liable for the waste that they generate

TREATMENT

On-site treatment where appropriate

Decontamination

Incineration

Neutralization of acids and bases

EMERGENCY AND CONTINGENCY PLANNING

Procedures for exposures, accidents, and spills

REVIEW AND REVISION

Frequently during implementation period and at least annually

Revisions and updates

Training programs include:
- Knowledge of federal, state, and local regulations that may apply
- The cost of HW procedures
- Cost and benefit analysis of waste disposal methods and alternatives
- Requirements and habits of waste generation of the laboratory

10.3.1 TRAINING PROGRAM IMPLEMENTATION

- All personnel should have prior training in the relevant standards such as the Hazard Communication, Bloodborne Pathogen, Formaldehyde, and Occupational Exposure to Hazardous Chemicals in Laboratories standards.
- All personnel must receive training and education in the risks associated with all types of waste, whether regulated or not.
- All personnel who handle hazardous or infectious waste must be trained when programs are implemented, prior to job assignment, when a process or procedure is changed, and at least annually thereafter.
- All personnel must be trained in the existence and location of the laboratory plan(s). Employees must be trained in the existence of applicable federal regulations and a copy of each regulation is made available to them.
- Training and continuing education must emphasize injury prevention, treatment, and emergency procedures. Training must also include incident reporting and follow-up procedures.
- Training must include the potential physical and health hazards of work areas and appropriate precautions for personnel protection.
- PPE requirements must be part of the training program. The use of gloves, gowns, coats, respirators, eye and facial protection, and foot coverings are also part of the instruction.
- All personnel should be trained in emergency or contingency plans and their applicable role in this plan.

10.3.2 SPECIAL DUTIES REGARDING SPILLS AND OTHER RELEASES

Personnel who may potentially respond to a release of hazardous substances must have special training. Contingency plans should be made to clean up small spills and should include the following procedures:
- Contain the spill
- Prevent personnel exposure
- Decontaminate

Larger spills may require facility emergency response team or local HAZMAT team of specially trained personnel.[1]

10.3.3 PROCEDURES REQUIRING PRIOR APPROVAL

- Define circumstances under which training and prior approval is necessary for a particular operation, activity, or procedure such as solvent distillation recovery and treatment of hazardous chemicals. (See also Figure 4.3 for a sample prior approval documentation form.)
- Appropriate training and supervision is required before prior approval is given.

10.3.4 SUPERVISOR RESPONSIBILITIES

The supervisor:
- Must be knowledgeable about waste management operations.

- Must apply effective purchasing strategies such as quantity control of material purchased.
- Must investigate and apply all options for in-house waste handling.
- Must maintain and enforce waste management procedures.

10.3.5 TRAINING EVALUATION AND MAINTENANCE

- The training program and documentation must be reviewed at least annually.
- Training must include all personnel involved in generation or handling of hazardous materials.
- Personnel must be trained in new procedures and updates as appropriate.
- Emergency response and special duty training must be given.
- Training on PPE, including respirators, must be given.
- Training in spills and eyewash station use and safety showers must be given.
- Posters, signs, and labels are used and training given for their meanings.

10.4 CATEGORIES OF LABORATORY WASTE[1]

10.4.1 CHEMICAL WASTE

Chemical waste is defined as (1) regulated waste and (2) unregulated waste that poses a threat to the environment or health; for example, any chemical waste that is ignitable, corrosive, reactive, or toxic. Obviously this list is extensive and it will be necessary to make individual assessments of chemicals to be considered. Consult the MSDS and other chemical-specific information.

It is important to note that the EPA principally addresses industrial waste streams and does not cover some laboratory chemical waste. Many laboratory wastes are nevertheless very hazardous and deserve special precautions. Also, do not forget that many states define toxicity more broadly than does the EPA and have additional laboratory chemical wastes regulations.

Have you ever heard the term "mad as a hatter" or know of the character in the classic *Alice in Wonderland* called the Mad Hatter? Do you know where the terms come from? Early workers in hat manufacturing used mercuric chloride solutions to cure the felt in the hats! Mercuric chloride is a violent poison. Knowledge and identification of the health hazards have multiplied and cannot be overstated.

10.4.1 A PROPERTIES OF CHEMICAL WASTE

Ignitability:
- Manifest and other report Identification No. DOO1 (Consult CFR 40 [261.21] for details of this class.)
- Flash point of <60°C or has some characteristic that has potential to cause fire
- Flammable liquids, including organic solvents (acetone, alcohol, toluene, xylene)
- Flammable gases, including hydrogen, silane, butane
- Oxidizers, such as nitrate salts and peroxides

- The EPA regulates organic solvents that are listed separately in CFR 40, Parts F, U, and P. Waste Identification Nos. 5001-5005 describe these solvents.

Corrosivity: Chemical waste substances have the capacity to corrode steel. (Described in detail in CFR 40 [261.22].) Examples include mineral acids—sulfuric, hydrochloric, and phosphoric—and bases such as ammonium hydroxide.

Reactivity: Chemical wastes are defined as follows:
- Any unstable substance that will readily undergo a violent change
- Reacts violently with water—potassium, sodium, other alkali metals
- Capable of detonation, such as explosives, dry picric acid, others that contain peroxides.
- Wastes that generate toxic gas, vapor or fumes, cyanide, or sulfuric solutions

Toxicity: There are two ways to identify toxicity in a waste. (1) Leachate Toxicity (Toxic Constituent Leachate Procedure [TCLP])—Identifies liquids that drain through or form waste containing toxic metals, pesticides, or certain other chemicals. (2) Lists of HW (P- and U- lists)—Letters refer to the identification number. Lists commercial chemical product and wastes from the cleanup of spills from these materials. (P-lists indicate "acute hazardous" waste.)

10.4.1 B SAFE CHEMICAL HANDLING[1]

Table 10.3 lists the chemicals that require safe HW disposal. Safe chemical handling includes the following:

Waste Segregation:
- Dilution of HW does not remove it from regulation, even if the waste mixture no longer has hazardous characteristics. The entire diluted mixture is now considered hazardous and is regulated.
- HW must be collected, transported, stored, and disposed of separately (segregated) from other waste.
- Waste solvents (if compatible) may be collected in one container. However, organic solvents may need individual collection for disposal purposes.

Engineering Controls:
- Ventilated storage room and nonventilated chemical storage cabinets
- Containment—(1) Devices to contain at least 10% of the volume of the containers or the volume of the largest of the containers (whichever is larger); (2) bench tops in laboratories can use high-walled trays; (3) large liquid containers in accumulation areas should be raised so if there is a spill or leak, the liquid does not contaminate the container
- Security regarding hazardous waste—(1) Safeguards are necessary to prevent access by unauthorized personnel in HW areas (generated, accumulated, or stored); (2) warning signs are recommended.
- Fire protection—(1) Appropriate containers and storage cabinets, explosion release doors; (2) grounded metal flammable liquid containers, fire suppression system; (3) appropriate fire extinguishers and alarm systems. (Consult NFPA 405 and 30 for additional details.)

- Physical facilities—Space for safe generation, storage and disposal procedures, aisle space for safe access, transport, and exit

Work Practices:
- Work practices regarding HW supplement, not substitute, proper engineering controls
- Work practices to minimize contamination of equipment, work surfaces, and PPE
- Work practice controls to ensure safe procedures will be used wherever possible
- Training in use of engineering controls, PPE, and protective devices is provided.
- Workers must inform management of unsafe working conditions.

Packaging and Labeling: Specific requirements for packaging and labeling of chemical waste are mandated for the point of generation, during handling, accumulation, and on-site storage and include:
- Collecting waste in containers compatible with waste type such as chemically resistant plastics for solvents and glass for mineral acids (sulfuric, hydro-chloric, and phosphoric acid)
- "Hazardous waste" label or marking
- Container tightly capped at all times

Table 10.3 CHEMICALS REQUIRING HAZARDOUS WASTE DISPOSAL

ORGANIC | | | INORGANIC

CHEMICALS

Acetone	1,2,dichloromethane	Polyethylene glycol	Ferric chloride	
Acetonitrile	Ethyl acetate	Ponceau S dye	Ferric cyanide	
Basic fuchsin	Ethylene dichloride	Pyridine	Potassium cyanide	
Benzidine (carcinogen)	Ethylene hydrochloride	Sodium acetate	Potassium permanganate	
Chloroform (carcinogen)	Ethylene glycol monoethyl ether	Trichloracetic acid	Silver nitrate	
Chromotrope	Hexane	Uranyl nitrate	Sodium azide (inactivated)	
Cyclohexane	Osmium tetroxide		Sodium nitrate	

ACIDS

Acetic acid	Ferric chloride	Silver nitrate
Tetrahydrofuran	Ferric cyanide	Sodium azide
Thiourea	Potassium cyanide	(inactivated)
Toluene	Potassium permanganate	

ALCOHOL DRUM | | BASE

Isoamyl alcohol	Ammonium hydroxide
Methanol	Sodium carbonate
Methylene chloride	Sodium hydroxide
N-Butyl alcohol	

- When shipped, must be packaged, labeled, marked with Department of Transportation (DOT) requirements.
- HW must have an additional special label (CFR 40 [262.32]).

PPE: Minimum requirements (particularly transfer procedures) must include:
- Goggles or face shields (regular or safety glasses are not appropriate for transfer procedures)
- Apron or laboratory coat
- Proper gloves
- Respirator used for volatile hazardous materials outside of fume hood

10.4.2 INFECTIOUS WASTE

Infectious waste includes (1) regulated waste as defined under the Bloodborne Pathogen Standard and (2) regulated medical waste (except unused sharps). Examples include cultures or stocks of infectious agents and associated biologicals, pathological waste, human blood and blood products, contaminated sharps, contaminated animal waste, isolation wastes, and any waste capable of producing infectious disease.

No actual disease transmission from public exposures to laboratory waste has been reported as of this writing. In fact, household waste may actually contain more pathogens. However, laboratories must consider the health and environmental problems associated with infectious waste handling, treatment, and disposal. The risk of disease transmission is greatest at the point of origin, thus making infectious waste a primary occupational hazard for health care workers. At least 90% of the states regulate infectious waste as waste that is capable of producing infectious disease.[3] Tables 10.4 and 10.5 list the categories of infectious waste as defined by the EPA and guidelines for an infectious waste management program, respectively.

10.4.2 A HANDLING OF INFECTIOUS WASTE

PPE:
- Use utility gloves—puncture and water resistant.
- Use barrier protective clothing.

Labeling:
- Place directly into plastic bags/containers clearly identifiable as infectious waste.
- Display biohazard symbol or use a red bag.
- Sharps containers must be labeled as biohazard even if they are placed in another primary disposal container.
- All untreated (infectious) containers must have biohazard warnings.

Segregation of Infectious Waste:
- Use color-coded or clearly marked containers.
- Separate uncontaminated materials from contaminated materials in each area for dramatic cost savings in disposal.
- Segregate infectious waste by treatment method as follows:
  - High water content—Incineration
  - High plastic content—Inappropriate for hospital incinerators (disposal service)
  - Autoclave—Microbiological materials

- Red bag materials—Disposal costs for red-bagged contaminated waste for an average outpatient clinic environment including the laboratory service can easily average $15,000 per year. Random audits of the waste deposited in red bags demonstrate that much of the waste can actually be classified as noninfectious waste. With operating costs spiraling, it is prudent for laboratories to review their waste disposal procedures and strive to reduce the amount of waste deposited into these red bag containers. Unless a significant amount of blood is visible, noninfectious materials do not need to be placed in a red bag, such as gloves that are not contaminated, eg, those used for chemicals or general purpose; blood-spotted bandages; Band-Aids; gauze or sponges; slightly soiled table or bench paper; used cotton swabs; tongue

Table 10.4 CATEGORIES OF INFECTIOUS WASTE

Pathological Waste	Wet tissues, organs, body parts, blood and body fluids removed during surgery, autopsy, and biopsy
Contaminated sharps	Contaminated hypodermic needles, syringes, scalpel blades, pasteur pipets, broken glass, used cover slips, used glass slides
Human blood and blood products	Waste blood, serum, plasma, and other blood components
Cultures and stocks of infectious agents	Specimens from medical and pathology laboratories and associated biologicals
Contaminated animal waste	Contaminated animal carcasses, body parts, and bedding of animals that were known to have been exposed to infectious disease
Isolation wastes	Blood, excretion, exudates, and secretions from patients with highly communicable disease

(From Environmental Protection Agency Guide for Infectious Waste Management, *1986)*

Table 10.5 GUIDELINES FOR AN INFECTIOUS WASTE MANAGEMENT PROGRAM

Designate a program coordinator or administrator.

Define infectious waste in the laboratory.

Define waste generating areas or sections of the laboratory.

Define waste composition and quantities generated.

Develop waste reduction policies/strategies.

Develop procedures and work practices to segregate, package, transport, store, on- and off-site treatment, and disposal of infectious waste.

Provide for review and quality assurance procedures.

Provide waste management training that includes emergency and contingency planning and appropriate safety programs.

Establish documentation policies and files for manifests, records of training and all other documentation pertinent to infectious waste management.

depressors; intravenous tubing; and hemocult cards. OSHA-defined regulated waste includes liquid or semiliquid blood or other potentially infectious materials (OPIM); contaminated items that would release blood or OPIM in a liquid or semiliquid state if compressed; items that are caked with dried blood or OPIM and are capable of releasing these materials during handling; contaminated sharps; and pathological and microbiological waste containing blood or OPIM.

Materials that should be placed in red bags include:
- Blood covered or grossly contaminated gloves
- Bandages soaked with blood or body fluids
- Blood-soaked Band-Aids, gauzes, or sponges
- Grossly contaminated table or bench paper with blood or body fluids
- Grossly contaminated Pap brushes
- Plastic centrifuge tubes and wound packing

10.4.2 B TREATMENT OF INFECTIOUS WASTE

The potential of diseases caused by infectious waste is usually reduced or eliminated by steam sterilization or incineration. A number of other methods (thermal inactivation, gas-vapor sterilization, chemical disinfection, etc) may be used, but for the purposes of this text, it is important to understand that decontamination is the standard goal of treatment. Reduction of pathologic microorganisms to a level below that which is necessary to transmit disease (decontamination), rather than elimination (sterilization), is adequate treat-ment (NCCLS).[1]

Chemical disinfection warrants specific attention because it is appropriate for treating certain liquid wastes or surfaces and may be particularly appropriate for many situations in the laboratory. The EPA considers chemical treatment as a disinfecting process, not a sterilizing process. Chemicals frequently used for disinfection include: (1) acids, alkalis, and aldehydes; (2) alcohols; (3) hydrogen peroxide; and (4) ammonium compounds.

Storage:
- Store for as brief a time as possible.
- Store in secure protected areas.

Transportation:
- Use appropriate, clearly labeled carts that are disinfected frequently.
- Avoid unnecessary personnel or patient exposure.
- Use no mechanical devices that could compromise containers.

Disposal Options: Treatment and disposal of infectious waste involves complex methodology and highly regulated mandates. Consult specific guidelines for these procedures which include on-site technologies and equipment for treatment and disposal as well as off-site disposal issues.

Incineration:
- Particularly advantageous for pathologic waste and sharps.

- Some local/regional regulations require strict incinerator procedures for hospitals.
- Burning plastics or multiple hazards with antineoplastic agents may require special considerations.
- Regional incinerators, shared by several facilities, may be an option and highly cost-effective.

Sanitary Sewers: If disposal of blood and body fluids into drains is allowed (check local health codes)
- Avoid splashes while decanting material into sink.
- Do not run water while decanting blood or body fluids into drain, then follow with copious amounts of water.
- Wear facial protection, waterproof aprons, gloves, and laboratory coats.
- Disposal sinks are not to be used for handwashing.

Emergency and Contingency Planning:
- Prevent sudden or accidental release of HW and the possibility of fire or explosion with precautions such as providing alarm systems, fire extinguishers, hoses, and automatic sprinklers.
- Make continency plans for medical treatment in case of emergencies such as accidents.
- Provide local fire, police, and hospital officials with information regarding the types of waste handled.
- Emergency phone numbers and locations of emergency equipment must be posted near telephones, and all employees must know proper waste handling and emergency procedures.
- An employee must be designated to act as emergency coordinator to ensure that procedures are carried out in the event of an emergency. The chemical hygiene officer may fill this role within a laboratory, while larger facilities may have institution spill or emergency teams in place, including an emergency coordinator on a facility-wide basis. (See also Table 4.3 and Table 6.2.)

10.4.3 RADIOACTIVE WASTE

Radioactive waste is generated from use of radioactive material. Examples include any solid, liquid, or gas emitting radiation. Glass, plastic, paper, soluble liquids, mixed insoluble liquids, urine, feces, blood, tissue, animal carcasses, cell culture dishes, and gases. Does not include sound or radio waves or visible or ultraviolet light, including lasers and diathermy units.

10.4.4 SHARPS

Sharps include wastes that can puncture and unused sharps, such as hypodermic needles, syringes, scalpel blades, lancets, capillary tubes, broken pipettes, glassware, broken blood tubes, broken culture dishes, slides, coverslips, wooden applicator sticks, and any object that can penetrate the skin. Because of the multiple hazards (whether contaminated or not), a waste management program should be prepared specifically for the handling, treatment, and disposal of sharps.

Management of sharps should include the following:
- Prevent injury from puncture or laceration.
- Prevent transmission of disease.
- Render needles and syringes useless before disposal.
- Render all sharps unrecognizable before disposal.
- Segregate all sharps (contaminated or not) from other waste materials.
- Label untreated sharps containers with warning words "infectious waste," medical waste, or biohazard symbol or red containers.
- Autoclave or incinerate. Destruction of sharps by incineration is the most commonly used method. These procedures are highly technical and highly regulated aspects of infectious waste management. Consult complete guidelines for detailed information.
- Use universal precautions.
- Minimize exposures.
- Replace glass or plastic pipettes with cannulas or plastic-tipped pipettes.
- Use similar replacement or elimination methods to reduce sharps.
- Package in sturdy corrugated fiberboxes with addition of absorbent material to absorb hazardous biological fluids and enhance incineration (engineering method).
- Place needles and blades in readily accessible "sharps containers."
- Decontaminate (autoclave) sharps containers before final disposal.

10.4.5 NHW

The RCRA defines solid waste as all solid, liquid, and gaseous waste that is not a mixture of sanitary sewerage. Hazardous chemical waste is considered a subset of solid waste and includes waste not included in the previously listed groups. NHW includes solid waste, sanitary sewerage, air emissions not considered to be infectious, radioactive waste, sharps, or chemically hazardous waste. NHW must be handled, managed, and disposed of properly because shattered plastics, some powders, or staples can cause injury if not properly disposed of and also are aesthetically unpleasant to the environment. Examples include any waste not known to pose substantial hazards, or present potential hazards, to human health or the environment.

10.4.5 A MANAGEMENT OF NHW
- *Reducing Generation of Waste*: Switch from disposable to durable goods where appropriate; reuse items that can be cleaned and sterilized.
- *Recycling*: Paper, glass, and other biodegradable organic materials.
- *Incineration*: Reduces volume of waste by 90%. However, the Clean Air Act may reduce the feasibility of incineration in some instances.
- *Segregation* methods are more and more frequently required by municipalities.
- *Liquid* NHW is disposed of in the waste water system or septic tank.

10.5 STORAGE OF LABORATORY WASTE[1]

10.5.1 CLASSIFICATIONS OF "GENERATORS"

EPA regulations are different depending on amounts of waste generated per month. The term "small quantity generator" is used to identify facilities producing more than 100 kg (220 lb) per month but less than 1000 kg (2200 lb) per month of acute HW.[4] Because the term "generator" is frequently used generically (as in this text), some states use the term "large quantity generator" to identify the most stringently regulated generation category. With respect to health care and medical facilities, few are considered to be "large quantity generators," most are classified as "small quantity generators." Table 10.6 lists the differences between the different categories of waste generators.

10.5.2 ACUTE HAZARDOUS WASTE
- Some wastes are considered to be acutely hazardous. The EPA has determined these wastes to be so dangerous in small amounts that they are regulated the same way as are large amounts of other hazardous waste.
- Generation of more than 1 kg per month (even if only one time) can require that additional criteria be met.

Table 10.6 CATEGORIES OF HAZARDOUS WASTE GENERATORS*[4]

MINIMUM GENERATORS	100-1000 KG PER MONTH	≥1000 KG PER MONTH
Conditionally exempt small quantity generator producing ≤100 kg (about 220 lb or 25 gallons) of hazardous waste and ≤1 kg (about 2.2 lbs) of acutely hazardous waste in any calendar month	Generators of >100 kg and <1000 kg (220-2200 lb or 25-300 gallons) of hazardous waste and ≤1 kg of acutely hazardous waste per month	≥1000 kg (about 2200 lb or 300 gallons) of hazardous waste or >1 kg of acutely hazardous waste in a month
Identify all hazardous waste generated. Send waste to a hazardous facility or landfill or other facility approved by the state for industrial or municipal wastes. Never accumulate >1000 kg of hazardous waste on your property (if you do, you become subject to all the requirements applicable to the 100-1000 kg-per-month generators).	Comply with the 1986 rules for managing hazardous waste, including accumulation, treatment, storage, and disposal requirements.	Comply with all applicable hazardous waste management requirements.

*1 barrel = about 200 kg of hazardous waste (or about one 55-gallon drum)

- It is important to dispose of waste regularly to avoid overaccumulation.
- Conditionally exempt small quantity generator is one who generates less than 100 kg of HW per month and less than 1 kg of acute HW per month.

10.5.3 STORAGE REQUIREMENTS

Requirements for small quantity generators include the following:
- Accumulation of no more than 6000 kg (thirty 55-gallon drums) of HW in any 180-day period (6 months).
- If transported more than 200 miles, time limit is extended to 290 days (9 months).

Requirements for conditionally exempt small quantity generators (most laboratories) are as follows:
- No time limit for storage
- Can store no more than 1000 kg (five 55-gallon drums) at one time

If stored in containers:
- Clearly mark each container with the words "Hazardous Waste" and the date collection of waste was begun in that container.
- Keep containers in good condition, free of leaks.
- Do not use a container, if it may rupture, leak, corrode, or fail.
- Keep containers closed except when filling or emptying.
- Inspect containers for leakage or corrosion every week.
- Make sure that reactive or ignitable wastes are stored as far as possible from the facility property line so as to create a buffer zone in case of an accident.
- Never store those wastes together that would react to cause fire, leaks, or other releases.
- Make sure that stored waste is taken off-site or treated on-site within 180 days.

If stored in tanks, consult the EPA for complete details.

10.6 TRANSPORTATION OF WASTE

It is vital that transportation of wastes follow EPA and DOT requirements and mandates. Most institutions find it desirable to contract a commercial waste (HW) transporter. Consult the complete *NCCLS Guidelines* for detailed information on selection of a commercial transporter.[1]

10.6.1 EPA IDENTIFICATION NUMBER

Laboratories, including all small quantity generators are required to have an EPA identification number. Call your state agency or EPA regional office to get a notification form. Fill out the form, sign it, and send it to the appropriate HW authority for your state. This is the identification number only, not the permit. (See also 10.7.) Also required is the EPA Notification of Hazardous Waste Activity Form (8700-12). Exempt small quantity generators, however, are not required to get an identification number.

10.6.2 MANIFEST

The EPA requires waste tracking "from cradle to the grave." Manifests:
- Identify generator, transporter, and destination of waste.
- Describe the waste and quantity.
- Make a copy for the generator when shipped and a copy to ensure that it arrived.
- Track and assign liability.
- Keep records well during the mandated 3-year period.

10.6.3 DOT REGULATIONS

- Use approved packaging and precautionary labeling with placard on vehicle.
- Lab packs with smaller waste containers inside may be metal or plastic, with plastic used for incineration.
- Use bulk solvent drums of 55-gallon size.

10.7 TREATMENT AND DISPOSAL METHODS

Figure 10.2 is a form that may be used to document on-site treatment procedures.

10.7.1 CONCERNS

- Future liability and occupational and environmental risks
- Facilitates self-reliance and cost.

10.7.2 UNKNOWN WASTE

- Illegible, deteriorated, or missing labels
- Follow prudent practices of chemical identification.

10.7.3 IN-LABORATORY NEUTRALIZATION

- Simple or elementary neutralization, such as mineral acid neutralization, is an EPA-exempt treatment; however, some states may be more restrictive.
- There are a number of approved procedures for treatment and disposal of hazardous chemicals. Before engaging in any disposal or neutralization procedure, make sure you understand and follow prescribed practices.

10.7.4 IN-LABORATORY REDUCTION

- In-laboratory treatment of HW requires EPA permit or state license; exceptions are neutralization and totally enclosed treatment facilities, which includes most laboratories.
- Nuclear Regulatory Commission describes in-laboratory reduction methods.
- Inexpensive disposal options exist for small amounts.
- Purchase small quantities—only as necessary.
- Use appropriate substitutes, xylene, formalin. Remember substitutes may only be "safer" but not necessarily "nontoxic" and many are considered to be HW. Change solutions when necessary.

10.7.5 COMMERCIAL DISPOSAL AND OTHERS

- Incineration or fuel blending
- Certain wastes are barred from landfills.
- For disposal of potentially explosive wastes, use police bomb squads.
- Recycle mercury (see 4.6.6) and other metals.
- Use commercial solvent recyclers if on-site recycling is not available.

Figure 10.2   SAMPLE ON-SITE TREATMENT PROCEDURE FORM FOR WASTE MANAGEMENT
SYSTEM

Date _____   Laboratory Section _____

Waste Category : [ ] Chemical   [ ] Infectious [ ] Sharps [ ] Nonhazardous

Specific material to be treated : _____

Type of On-Site Treatment:

[ ]   Neutralization

[ ]   Recycling

[ ]   In-Laboratory Reduction

[ ]   Commercial Disposal Guidelines

Procedure or Process Discription:

_____

_____

_____

Process/Procedure Reference:

_____

_____

_____

Procedure/Process Authorized by _____   Date _____

Review and Evaluation Schedule _____

_____

10.7.6 SANITARY SEWER SYSTEMS

If approved by local sanitation district, it may be acceptable to dispose of dilute solutions of some toxic metals or other HW. (See CFR 40-261.4.) Some facilities have mixing tanks designed to neutralize and dilute waste acids. Check with facility for existence of such tanks and obtain training for proper use.

10.8 METHODS OF WASTE MINIMIZATION[1,2]

Waste minimization is an essential part of a facility waste management program. A formal waste minimization program is not a requirement for conditionally exempt small quantity generators but they must demonstrate good faith effort.

10.8.1 ON-SITE RECYCLING

- Reclamation of laboratory solvents and fixatives has become a cost-effective and efficient method of on-site recycling. Xylene, alcohol, formalin, as well as number of solvent substitutes may be successfully recovered and recycled by most laboratories, thereby not only providing a dramatic reduction of HW, but also demonstrating a sizable economic advantage by reducing the amount of reagents purchased (see also 10.2).
- Recycle cans, paper, and other solid materials.
- Redistribute chemical surplus to other areas or sections of the laboratory.
- Develop chemical banks for access by other laboratory areas or sections.

10.8.2 RECOVERY

There are several recovery units as well as methods developed for the use of waste solvent for fuels. However, this technology may not be practical or cost-effective for most laboratory environments.

10.9 SUMMARY[4]

The most important concepts of waste management include the following:

Reduce the amount of HW.
- Do not mix NHW with HW because the entire contents become hazardous.
- Avoid mixing several different HWs. Doing so may make recycling difficult, if not impossible, or make disposal more expensive.
- Avoid spills or leaks of hazardous products. (The materials used to clean up such spills or leaks are also considered hazardous.)
- Make sure the original containers of HW are completely empty before throwing them away. Use all of the product.
- Avoid using more of the hazardous material than needed.
- Reducing HW means saving money and reducing disposal costs and liabilities.

Table 10.7 is a summarizing list of materials that are counted as HW and those that are not.

Conduct self-inspections. This is the best way to prepare for inspections. The following basic checklist can serve as guide and aid in developing a facility handbook:

[ ] Do you have documentation on the amounts and kinds of HW you generate, and how do you determine that they are hazardous?

[ ] Do you have an EPA identification number?

[ ] Do you ship waste off-site? If so, by which hauler and to which designated HW management facility?

[ ] Do you have copies of all manifests used to ship your HW off-site? Are they filled out correctly? Have they been signed by the designated facility?

[ ] Is your HW stored in the proper containers?

[ ] Are the containers properly dated and marked?

[ ] Have you designated an emergency coordinator?

[ ] Have you posted emergency telephone numbers and the location of emergency equipment?

[ ] Are employees thoroughly familiar with proper waste handling and emergency procedures?

[ ] Do you understand that you may need to contact the National Response Center (usually industrial applications)?

Table 10.7 WHAT TO COUNT AS HAZARDOUS WASTE[4]

HAZARDOUS WASTE

Accumulated on site for any period prior to management

Packaged and transported off-site

Placed directly in a regulated on-site treatment or disposal unit

Generated as still bottoms or sludges and removed from product storage tanks

WASTES NOT COUNTED AS HAZARDOUS

Wastes specifically exempted, such as oil not mixed with hazardous waste

May be left in the bottom of containers that have been completely emptied through conventional means, by pouring or pumping (containers used for acute hazardous waste must be thoroughly cleaned)

Left as residue in the bottom of storage tanks if the residue is not removed from the product tank

Reclaimed continuously on-site without storing, such as solvents

Managed in an elementary neutralization unit (a regulated tank, container, or transport vehicle designed to contain and neutralize corrosive wastes), a totally enclosed treatment unit, or a wastewater treatment unit

Discharged directly to a publicly owned treatment works (facility usually owned by the city, county, or state to treat industrial and domestic sewage for disposal) without being stored or accumulated first, in compliance with the Clean Water Act

Already used once during the month and treated on-site or reclaimed in some manner and used again

Cooperate with state and local inspectors. Inspectors serve as an excellent source of information on recordkeeping, manifests, and safety requirements specific to a facility. Inspections should be an opportunity to identify and correct problems.

Call your state HW management agency or the EPA with any questions.

10.10 REFERENCES

1. National Committee for Clinical Laboratory Standards. *Clinical Laboratory Waste Management: Approved Guidelines.* Villanova, Pa: National Committee for Clinical Laboratory;1994. Document GP5-A 19085.
2. Chovit K, Rhodes D. Effective hazardous waste management helps generators, reduces cost. *Occup Health Saf.* April 1994:25-29.
3. Watson L. Handling waste. *Adv Administr Lab.* March-April 1993:15-19.
4. US Department of Environmental Protection Agency. *Understanding the Small Quantity Generator Hazardous Waste Rules: A Handbook for Small Business.* Washington, DC: US EPA; 1986.

10.10.1 ADDITIONAL READINGS

Burns J. Turning a problem into a product. *Mod Healthcare Facilities Management.* August 1991:17-19.

Crookham J. Consumer awareness in the laboratory. Presented at the National Society for Histotechnology Meeting; Philadelphia, Pa; October 8, 1993.

Crookham J, Dapson R. Drain disposal of laboratory chemicals. *Lipshaw Lableader.* 1992;7(2):3-7.

Grushka M. Recycling xylene saves money and the environment. *Med Lab Observer.* July 1991:55-60.

Miller H. Administration of hazardous waste reduces problems of compliance. *Occup Health Saf.* November 1987.

Miller L. Coast-to-coast state waste regulations. *Lab Animal.* September 1991:20-25.

Appendix

A1 HEALTH AND SAFETY COMPLIANCE EVALUATION TESTS

One of the best methods of testing a program for regulatory compliance is to answer specific questions regarding the program format. The Health and Safety Compliance Evaluation is provided so that the laboratory can test itself regarding compliance with the Occupational Safety and Health Administration (OSHA) standards covered in this text. Evaluation of programs for strengths and weaknesses is readily apparent on completion of this testing. Questions are provided concerning the Hazard Communication Standard, Occupational Exposures to Hazardous Chemicals in Laboratories, the Formaldehyde Standard, and the Bloodborne Pathogen Standard. Also provided are questions that represent a "mock inspection" such as those given by the College of American Pathologists (CAP).

A1.1 THE HAZARD COMMUNICATION STANDARD (THE RIGHT-TO-KNOW LAW)

1. Have notices been posted telling employees that they have the right to know? [ ]
2. Has an inventory of hazardous substances been made? Is it updated regularly? [ ]
3. Do all hazardous substances, chemicals, and reagents have appropriate labeling? [ ]
   Chemical manufacturers [ ]
   Identity of the hazardous material? [ ]
   Appropriate hazard warnings? [ ]
   Name and address of the manufacturer? [ ]
   Emergency phone number? [ ]
   Expiration date and lot number? [ ]
   In-house chemical not in original container [ ]
      Identity of hazardous chemical? [ ]
      Route of entry? [ ]
      Health hazard? [ ]
      Physical hazard? [ ]
      Target organ affected by substance? [ ]
4. Are MSDSs maintained on all hazardous substances? [ ]
5. Does information documented (MSDS) on all hazardous substances include:
      Product and ID number? [ ]
      Hazardous ingredients? [ ]
      Fire and explosion information? [ ]
      Physical data? [ ]
      Health hazards? [ ]
      Reactivity? [ ]
      Protective equipment? [ ]
      Spill and leak information? [ ]
      Handling and storage information? [ ]
      Special information as appropriate? [ ]
6. Are MSDSs maintained in an orderly fashion and updated as new data are received while maintaining original information that may have been in place during certain employee coverage? [ ]
7. Has a program of training and education been established for all employees? [ ]
8. Does the training program educate and train employees in safe and proper handling of hazardous substances? [ ]
9. Is the training program given before initial assignment of work and annually thereafter? [ ]
10. Is this information updated as new data or information is received? [ ]
11. Do employees know that they may request information concerning any hazardous substance that they may work with? [ ]

12. Is there an employee request form for hazardous substance information? [ ]
13. Does the employee receive this information in writing? [ ]
    Within 3 working days? [ ]
14. Are all records of training, updates, employee requests, or significant incident reports maintained? [ ]

NOTE: The NFPA diamond is NOT required, but rather NFPA-type hazard warning systems are sufficient as long as all employees know the meanings of the hazard system used.

A1.2 OCCUPATIONAL EXPOSURES TO HAZARDOUS CHEMICALS IN LABORATORIES

1. Is there a designated chemical hygiene officer and do all employees know who this is and how he or she can be reached? [ ]
2. Does the laboratory use OSHA-regulated substances? [ ]
3. Have employers measured (monitored) their employees' exposure to regulated substances, such as formaldehyde, in the workplace? [ ]
4. If the exposure level is above the action level (AL) (or in the absence of an AL, the permissible exposure limit [PEL]) for an OSHA-regulated substance that has exposure monitoring and medical surveillance requirements, has a medical surveillance been established for the affected employee? [ ]
5 Does the use of hazardous chemicals meet the definition of laboratory use? [ ]
6. Are MSDSs in the work area for all hazardous materials? [ ]
7. Are MSDSs used by the employees? [ ]
8. If respirators are used, are they of proper type with the proper filter? [ ]
9. Are employees personally fitted for each respirator? [ ]
10. Are employees trained in the operation and use of respirators? [ ]
11. Is there a decontamination and maintenance procedure for respirators? [ ]
12. Do employees receive a medical examination if they are exposed to a hazardous material? [ ]
13. Are records maintained for each employee to monitor exposures, medical consultations, medical examination, test results, and written records? [ ]
14. Do employees have access to all training materials, monitoring records, exposure incidents, and medical records? [ ]

A1.2.1 THE CHEMICAL HYGIENE PLAN

1. Is there a written chemical hygiene plan capable of keeping the exposure levels below the PEL? [ ]
2. Do the employees have a written copy of the chemical hygiene plan or appropriate employee information packet? [ ]
3. Does the chemical hygiene plan detail handling of the hazardous material? [ ]
4. Is the complete chemical hygiene plan available to all personnel during their work hours? [ ]
5. Does the chemical hygiene plan implement engineering controls? [ ]
6. Does the chemical hygiene plan require measures to ensure proper performance of fume hoods and other engineering equipment? [ ]
7. Does the chemical hygiene plan outline which procedures require prior approval from the employer before implementation? [ ]
8. Is a prior approval form included in the chemical hygiene plan? [ ]
9. Is there a specific area designated for the use of hazardous materials? [ ]
10. Does the chemical hygiene plan outline procedures for the safe removal and disposal of contaminated waste? [ ]
11. Does the chemical hygiene plan detail decontamination procedures? [ ]
12. Does the employee review and evaluate the chemical hygiene plan at least annually for effectiveness and updating? [ ]

13. Does the plan include standard operating procedures for the use of hazardous substances? [ ]
14. Are there measures to ensure properly functioning equipment? [ ]
15. Is there an employee information and training program described and implemented? [ ]
16. Is there an employee review, effectiveness of program evaluation, and update of the program at least annually? [ ]
17. Are there records of training for all employees? [ ]
18. Are employees informed of:
    The contents of this standard? [ ]
    The location and availability of the plan? [ ]
    PELs for hazardous chemicals? [ ]
    Signs and symptoms associated with exposures? [ ]
    Location and availability of reference material? [ ]
    Methods to detect hazardous chemicals exposure? [ ]
    Physical and health hazards of chemicals? [ ]
    Methods of protection to avoid exposure? [ ]
    Understand terminology of the standard such as "laboratory scale" and " laboratory use"? [ ]
19. Do all employees:
    Understand the meaning and use of signage and labeling systems? [ ]
    Understand and be able to implement emergency procedures in case of a hazardous chemical spill? [ ]
20. Is appropriate personal protective equipment provided (PPE)? [ ]
21. Are there clearly written and established guidelines and procedures for use of personal protective equipment? [ ]
22. Are employees trained in the use of PPE? [ ]
23. Are employees informed of enforcement measures to ensure use of PPE? [ ]
24. Are there provisions for medical consultation and examinations? [ ]
25. Are there provisions for particularly hazardous chemical protection? [ ]
    Designated areas for use? [ ]
    Containment devices, like hoods? [ ]
    Safe waste removal? [ ]
    Decontamination procedures? [ ]
26. Are there established written procedures for general housekeeping and physical maintenance of the laboratory area? [ ]
27. Are appropriate safety and emergency equipment provided? [ ]
    Fire alarm? [ ]
    Eye wash stations? [ ]
    Fire extinguishers? [ ]
    Fire blanket? [ ]
    Chemical spill kits? [ ]
    Broom, dust pan, sharps containers? [ ]
    Safety shower? [ ]
28. Is personnel knowledgeable concerning the use of, procedure for, and location of:
    Fire alarm? [ ]
    Fire extinguishers and blanket? [ ]
    Safety showers and eyewash stations? [ ]
29. Are appropriate fire, spill, or other appropriate drills held regularly? [ ]
30. Are appropriate records and documentation maintained for:
    Safety/housekeeping inspections? [ ]

Preventive maintenance on all equipment?	[ ]
Accident or exposure incidents?	[ ]
Follow-up evaluations?	[ ]
Safety training programs?	[ ]
Fire and other emergency drills?	[ ]
Exposure monitoring results?	[ ]

31. Are emergency phone numbers, hospitals codes, and home phone numbers for key personnel posted? [ ]
32. Are original chemical container labels left intact? [ ]
33. Do all chemical containers have appropriate warning labels? [ ]
34. Is an explanation of hazard warning systems posted in a prominent location in the laboratory work area? [ ]
35. Are significant hazards throughout the laboratory clearly identified with symbols and writing including:
    Flammable liquid storage? [ ]
    Biological waste receptacles? [ ]
    Areas containing radioactive materials? [ ]
    Storage areas for strong alkalis or acids? [ ]
36. Is the location of safety equipment clearly marked and identified? [ ]
37. Does the laboratory participate in internal and external disaster drills? [ ]
38. Are there designated personnel for chemical spill response? [ ]
39. Are these designated personnel given initial training and retraining with regards to spill procedures? [ ]
40. With regard to the chemical hygiene program, are there written guidelines for the responsibilities of the chemical hygiene officer, responsibilities of the managers and supervisors, and the responsibilities of the laboratory personnel? [ ]

A1.3 THE FORMALDEHYDE STANDARD

1. Is there an established written program and procedures for the use, handling, and storage of formaldehyde in the laboratory? [ ]
2. Is there a statement of implementation for a formaldehyde safety program? [ ]
3. Is there a program of employee monitoring (task assessment) for each job classification for each workshift? [ ]
4. Is employee monitoring (task assessment) repeated each time there is a change in production, equipment, process, personnel, or control measures which may result in new or additional exposure to formaldehyde? [ ]
5. If there are areas in which the concentration of airborne formaldehyde may exceed the PEL or short-term exposure limit (STEL), do all entrances and accessways have signs bearing warning information? [ ]
6. When respirators are used, do these rules apply:
    Negative pressure respirators are used? [ ]
    Individual employee training the personal fitting of respirator to be used? [ ]
    Training and fitting repeated annually? [ ]
    Is this training documented? [ ]
    When used, chemical cartridges are replaced after 3 hours of service or at end of workshift? [ ]
    Is this procedure documented? [ ]
    Employees wash their faces to prevent skin irritation from respirator use? [ ]
    Are respirators maintained, cleaned, and checked for defects regularly? Is this procedure documented? [ ]
7. Are safety showers and eyewash stations readily available? [ ]

8.   Are there regular visual inspections to detect spills or leaks of formaldehyde?   [ ]
9.   Are these inspections documented?   [ ]
10.   Is there a specific spill clean-up procedure for formaldehyde?   [ ]
11.   Is there a complete medical surveillance program?   [ ]
12.   Is there a medical surveillance questionnaire given to each employee upon initial assignment and annually thereafter to determine the risk of the employee to formaldehyde? (Nonmandatory except in certain situations. See standard.)   [ ]
13.   Are there provisions for employee reassignment or retraining if employees become sensitive to formaldehyde exposure?   [ ]
14.   Is there an established exposure incident recording procedure?   [ ]
15.   Is there an established exposure incident follow-up and evaluation procedure to identify methods to prevent future incidents?   [ ]
16.   Is there a complete training program for all personnel?   [ ]
17.   Is it given at the time of initial assignment, annually, and whenever a new exposure to formaldehyde is introduced to the workplace?   [ ]
18.   Is it given at a level of understanding for the audience?   [ ]
19.   Does it explain the contents of the standard?   [ ]
20.   Does it explain the contents of the MSDS?   [ ]
21.   Does it give the purpose of and describe the medical surveillance program?   [ ]
22.   Does it describe the potential health hazards?   [ ]
23.   Does it describe the signs and symptoms of formaldehyde exposure?   [ ]
24.   Does it explain safe work practices for limiting exposure to formaldehyde in each job classification?   [ ]
25.   Does it describe the purpose, proper use of, and limitations of PPE?   [ ]
26.   Are there specific instructions for handling spills, emergencies, and clean-up procedures?   [ ]
27.   Is there an explanation of the importance of engineering and work practice controls for employee protection?   [ ]
      Is there necessary instruction in the use of these controls?   [ ]
28.   Is there a review of emergency procedures including the specific duties or assignments of each employee in the event of an emergency?   [ ]
29.   Are environmental monitoring records kept for 30 years?   [ ]
30.   Are medical records kept for the length of employment plus 30 years?   [ ]
31.   Are respirator fit records kept until replaced by a more recent record?   [ ]
32.   Has an estimate of total formaldehyde usage been made?   [ ]
33.   Are there established procedures for disposal of waste formaldehyde?   [ ]
34.   Have procedures and responsibilities been determined for movement of formaldehyde throughout a facility (surgery specimens, clinic specimens, doctors, offices)?   [ ]
35.   Has appropriate storage of formaldehyde been achieved?   [ ]
36.   Have appropriate hoods or effective ventilation been provided for high risk areas?   [ ]
37.   Are hoods and ventilation systems maintained and checked regularly for performance?   [ ]
      Is this documented?   [ ]

A1.4 THE BLOODBORNE PATHOGEN STANDARD

1.   Has training been given prior to beginning the job?   [ ]
2.   Is retraining or updates given as needed?   [ ]
3.   Has training been given by a qualified instructor?   [ ]
4.   Is the name of this instructor documented?   [ ]
5.   Was the instructor available for questions?   [ ]

6. Was the training given at the knowledge level of the audience?   [ ]
7. Is there a complete record of training?   [ ]
      Were pre/post tests given?   [ ]
8. Did the training include:
      An explanation of the contents of the law?   [ ]
      The compliance date of the program? (May 1992)   [ ]
      Prime targets of infection?   [ ]
      Proper use of PPE?   [ ]
      Work practices, such as handwashing?   [ ]
      Proper handling and disposal of sharps?   [ ]
      Use of engineering controls, such as hoods?   [ ]
      Immunization programs with vaccination?   [ ]
      Proper handling and disposal of contaminated waste?   [ ]
      Use of disinfectants and decontamination procedures?   [ ]
      Labeling, warning systems, and signs?
      General epidemiology and symptoms of bloodborne pathogen diseases?   [ ]
      Modes by which bloodborne pathogens are transmitted?   [ ]
9. Has an infection control plan been written?   [ ]
10. Does the infection control plan include:
      Task categories (job descriptions) of potential exposures?   [ ]
      A hazard inventory to determine potential exposure?
11. Have engineering controls been developed to minimize exposures?   [ ]
      Sharps containers?   [ ]
      Biocabinets?   [ ]
      Decontamination schedules?   [ ]
      Splash shields?   [ ]
      Maintenance schedules?   [ ]
12. Has PPE been furnished?   [ ]
      Gloves (latex, vinyl, hypoallergenic, utility, stainless steel mesh)?   [ ]
      Gowns, laboratory coats?   [ ]
      Goggles?   [ ]
      Full face shields?   [ ]
      Aprons?   [ ]
      Caps, shoe covers?   [ ]
      Respirators?   [ ]
13. Have work practices been established to minimize exposures?   [ ]
      Disinfection of workstations and instruments?   [ ]
      Disinfection of PPE?   [ ]
      Emphasis on handwashing?   [ ]
      Wearing closed, long sleeve, cuffed gowns, or coats?   [ ]
      Wearing and removing gloves?   [ ]
      Contamination control (telephones, computers, doorknobs)?   [ ]
      Glassware handling?   [ ]
      Contaminated waste disposal?   [ ]
      Housekeeping, laundry, and bench coverings?   [ ]
14. Does the plan contain recognition of exposure situations?   [ ]
15. Does the plan contain proper selection of PPE for exposure situations?   [ ]
16. Does the plan contain procedures for exposure situations?   [ ]
      Reporting procedures for exposure situations?   [ ]

Procedures for follow-up evaluation to prevent future incidents? [ ]

17. Does the plan contain information on hepatitis B virus (HBV) vaccination? [ ]
18. Does the plan contain documentation of vaccination or refusal of vaccination? [ ]
19. Does the plan contain emergency procedures, such as spills? [ ]
    Are appropriate spill kits available? [ ]
    Are appropriate clean-up instruments available, such as absorbent material,
    broom, dust pan, tongs? [ ]
20. Does the plan describe signs and labeling procedures? [ ]
    Are appropriate "biohazard" signs used? [ ]
    Are there signs to indicate PPE and/or removal of PPE, ie, before leaving laboratory? [ ]
    Are there designated "clean" and "dirty" sinks? [ ]
    Is laundry properly contained? [ ]
    Are laboratory coats close to work area? Are there laboratory coat hooks or hangers? [ ]
    Do personnel use gloves when handling laundry? [ ]
    Are secondary containers used where appropriate? [ ]
21. Are special requirements for HIV and HBV research laboratories written, if appropriate? [ ]
22. Are safety policies and procedures written? [ ]
23. Are safety policies posted in the autopsy suite? [ ]
24. Do the safety polices and procedures provide instructions for daily cleaning? [ ]
    Cleaning after autopsy? [ ]
    Proper handling of highly infectious material? [ ]
    Disposal of contaminated tissues? [ ]
25. Are personal protective provisions made for the examination of highly infectious cases? [ ]
    Masks? Respirators, if applicable? [ ]
    Gowns, laboratory coats, and aprons? [ ]
    Gloves (latex or vinyl, utility, and stainless steel mesh)? [ ]
    Shoe or foot coverings? [ ]
    Eye protection? [ ]
    Shields for full face? [ ]
26. Are there procedures for disinfection of nondisposable PPE? [ ]
    Aprons? [ ]
    Full face shields? [ ]
    Mesh and utility gloves? [ ]
    Respirators? [ ]
27. Are there procedures for disposal of disposable PPE? [ ]
    Masks, gloves, gowns, and aprons? [ ]
28. Is there proper disinfection after use of: [ ]
    Tables and work surfaces? [ ]
    Instruments? [ ]
    Pans and trays? [ ]
    Photographic equipment? [ ]
29. Are there written procedures for the special handling of cases of Creutzfeldt-Jacob syndrome
    and for patients who have died from undiagnosed encephalopathy? [ ]
30. Are formaldehyde and xylene vapor concentrations maintained at permissible concentrations? [ ]

A1.4.1 EVALUATING THE TRAINING AND EDUCATIONAL PROGRAM

1. Are the effective dates for compliance and explanation of the contents of the Bloodborne Pathogen
    Standard provided? [ ]

2. Is an instructor present for discussion and questions from participants? [ ]
3. Is the training evaluated with a program for review and discussion with instructors and employees? [ ]
4. Does the program include epidemiology, clinical symptoms, modes of transmission, and methods for prevention of HBV and HIV? [ ]
5. Does the program describe protective measures to be taken to prevent exposure? [ ]
6. Has a program been established for workers actually or potentially exposed to blood or body fluids? [ ]
7. When is the training program presented? [ ]
   New employee orientation? [ ]
   Annually? [ ]
   Updated as appropriate? [ ]
8. Does the training program cover:
   Universal precautions? [ ]
   PPE? [ ]
   Workplace practices to reduce and minimize exposures? [ ]
   Procedures for needle stick or physical exposure? [ ]
   Hepatitis B vaccination program? [ ]
9. Is the effectiveness of the program monitored by worker compliance with guidelines? [ ]
10. Does the program identify specific procedures to provide exposure protection such as PPE use? [ ]
11. Are appropriate facilities provided for compliance with workplace practices? [ ]
    Handwashing sinks? [ ]
    Needle disposal containers? [ ]
    Disinfectants? [ ]
12. Are specific workplace practice procedures established for:
    Handwashing? [ ]
    Handling sharp instruments? [ ]
    Blood or specimen spills? [ ]
    Disposal of contaminated materials? [ ]
    Decontamination of reusable materials? [ ]

A1.5 "MOCK" CAP INSPECTION

Questions are relevant to health and safety.
1. Do all personnel have access to all safety policies and procedures? [ ]
2. Are policies and procedures developed for documentation of all laboratory accidents resulting in property damage or involving spillage of hazardous materials? [ ]
3. Are policies and procedures developed for documentation of all occupational injuries or illnesses that require medical treatment, not just first aid? [ ]
4. Is there a program of follow-up evaluation of these incidents or accident reports to prevent reccurrence? [ ]
5. Is there an annual review and evaluation of the effectiveness of the chemical hygiene plan? [ ]
6. Are adequate safety policies and procedures established for:
   Fire prevention and control? [ ]
   Electrical safety? [ ]
   Hazardous chemical hazard control? [ ]
   Biohazard control? [ ]
   Hazardous waste disposal? [ ]
   Internal and external disaster preparedness? [ ]
   Radiation safety? [ ]
7. Are there periodic reviews of safe work practices? [ ]
   Are they documented? [ ]

8. If the laboratory does not have an automatic sprinkler system, is it separated from surrounding health care area by fire-resistive construction? [ ]

9. Are fire drills conducted quarterly? [ ]

10. Do all rooms have direct and unimpeded access to the hall or secondary exit? [ ]

11. Is the fire alarm, PA system, or fire bell audible in all sections of the laboratory? [ ]

12. Is there an established, appropriate evacuation plan? [ ]

13. Does this plan include handicapped individuals? [ ]

14. Is there an alarm system in or near the laboratory? [ ]

15. Are appropriate fire extinguishers available? [ ]

16. In areas that have 1-gallon flammable or combustibles, are there fire extinguishers for Class B (10:B) provided? [ ]

17. Are Class B fire extinguishers provided in areas with solvent fire hazards? [ ]

18. Are personnel instructed in the use of fire extinguishers? [ ]
    Is this training documented? [ ]

19. Are safety cans used instead of glass bottles for volumes of solvents more than 1 qt? (Unless purity requires glass, such as ether or pentane.) [ ]

20. Are flammable liquids properly stored? (5000 sq ft allows 60 gallons stored in safety cabinets; up to 25 gallons may be stored in safety can; up to 10 gallons may be stored in open shelves.) [ ]

21. Is there adequate ventilation for storage areas where volatile solvents are stored? [ ]

22. Are flammable or combustible liquids or gas cylinders kept well away from open flames or other heat sources? [ ]
    Away from open corridors or within exhaust hoods? [ ]

23. Are grounds used when flammables are decanted from large drum containers? [ ]

24. Are flammable-gas cylinders stored in an exclusive, separate, ventilated room or enclosure just for that purpose? [ ]

25. Is this area fire-resistant for at least 2 hours? (CO_2 is not flammable.) [ ]

26. Is there an eyewash station within 100 ft of every area where hazardous chemicals are used? [ ]

27. Is there documentation of the eyewash station being tested regularly? [ ]

28. Is PPE used when handling corrosive, flammable, and carcinogenic substances? [ ]

29. Are there procedures for monitoring and enforcement of personal protective equipment use? [ ]

30. Is there documentation for assuring proper functioning of all protective equipment, such as hoods, centrifuges, etc? [ ]

31. Are there bottle carriers for transport of all glass containers larger than 500 mL used for hazardous chemicals? [ ]

32. Are explicit instructions posted, supplies and equipment provided for emergency treatment of chemical splashes or major chemical spills and any resulting injuries? [ ]

33. Is there an emergency lighting system in the laboratory? [ ]

34. Are all fixed, electrical receptacles checked for polarity and proper grounding at least annually? [ ]
    Is this documented? [ ]

35. Are all instruments and appliances adequately grounded and checked for current leakage at least annually? [ ]
    Is this documented? [ ]

36. With regard to toxic and biological hazards:
    Is proper notification of personnel given? [ ]
    Are the types of hazards identified? [ ]
    Are precautions given if exposure occurs? [ ]
    Are restrictions (access) to certain hazardous areas given? [ ]
    Are certain personnel (susceptible to exposure) monitored? [ ]
    Is there a complete inventory of all hazardous materials? [ ]

37. Are all toxic chemicals (either bulk or concentrated forms) clearly labeled as to type of hazard and emergency actions? [ ]
38. Are there precautionary labels present on all containers of hazardous chemicals? [ ]
39. Are there warnings on all flammable liquids and combustibles listing Class I, II, IIIA? [ ]
40. Is there a written policy for universal precautions for bloodborne pathogens? [ ]
41. Is a copy of the proposed guideline Protection of Laboratory Workers from Infectious Disease transmitted by Blood and Tissue (NCCLS Document M29-A, Vol 7, No 9) available to all personnel? [ ]
    Is a copy of the OSHA Standard on Bloodborne Pathogens (29 CFR 1910:1030) available to all personnel? [ ]
42. Is appropriate PPE provided? [ ]
    Gloves, downs, masks, eye protection? [ ]
    Maintained in sanitary and reliable condition? [ ]
    In all technical areas where blood and body substances may be found? [ ]
43. Are gloves provided, readily available, and mandatory? (Mandatory for phlebotomists; exception is voluntary blood donor centers.) [ ]
44. Are all personnel instructed in:
    Proper use of gloves? [ ]
    Proper disposal of gloves? [ ]
    Need for properly fitting gloves? [ ]
    Replacing gloves if torn or contaminated? [ ]
    No washing or disinfecting of gloves for reuse? (Exceptions: utility and mesh) [ ]
45. Is training given to personnel reasonably expected to be exposed to body substances including:
    Precautionary measures? [ ]
    Epidemiology? [ ]
    Modes of transmission? [ ]
    Universal precautions? [ ]
    Work practices? [ ]
46. Are vaccinations for HBV offered to personnel who are reasonably expected to be exposed to body substances? [ ]
47. Is there documentation of vaccinations or declination of the hepatitis B vaccination? [ ]
48. Is there a policy for follow-up procedures for possible or known exposures to HIV or HBV? [ ]
49. Does it include:
    Testing of the source of exposure for HIV and HBV? (After consent is obtained?) [ ]
    Clinical and serological evaluation of the worker? [ ]
    Consideration of prophylaxis for acutely exposed personnel to HIV or HBV? [ ]
    Serologic status and informed consent of the worker? [ ]
50. Are smoking, eating, drinking, application of cosmetics or lip balm, manipulation of contact lenses and mouth pipetting prohibited in writing for all technical work areas? [ ]
51. Are all devices for sterilizing monitored for effectiveness of sterility under simulated use conditions? [ ]
52. With regard to needles, is there a written and informed policy that prohibits:
    Recapping needles? [ ]
    Bending of needles? [ ]
    Breaking of needles? [ ]
    Removing needles from disposable syringes? [ ]
    Otherwise manipulating needles by hand? [ ]
    Exception: Resheathing instruments or self-sheathing needles used to prevent recapping of needles by hand.

53. Are vacuum breakers (antisiphon) provided on water outlets where applicable? [ ]
54. Has documentation been made that each chemical in the laboratory has been evaluated for:
    Carcinogenic effect? [ ]
    Reproductive toxicity? [ ]
    Acute toxicity? [ ]
55. Are there policies and procedures for specific handling requirements for each hazardous chemical? [ ]
    Is there a procedure manual? [ ]
56. Do all workers have access to:
    MSDS? [ ]
    References for safe handling of chemicals with details? [ ]
    The chemical hygiene plan? [ ]
    A copy of OSHA's Occupational Exposures to Hazardous Chemicals in Laboratories
    (29 CFR 1910:1450)? [ ]
57. Is there evidence that the laboratory has reviewed real or potential hazardous waste, stages of disposal, transportation, final disposal, and local, state, and federal regulations to be sure they are in compliance? [ ]
58. Are methods of disposal of all solid or liquid waste in compliance with local, state, and federal agencies? [ ]
    Is this documented? [ ]
    Are manifests maintained? [ ]
59. Are all infectious wastes incinerated or appropriately decontaminated before being sent to sanitary landfills? [ ]
60. Are corrosive, ignitable, and toxic wastes disposed of safely and in properly labeled containers? [ ]
61. Are sterile syringes, needles, lancets, or other similar devices capable of transmitting infection used only once? [ ]
62. Are all waste sharps containers puncture-resistant? [ ]
    Easily accessible? [ ]
    Properly labeled? [ ]
    Leak-proof? [ ]
    Not overfilled? [ ]
    Closable? [ ]
63. Is each open automated tissue processor operated at least 5 feet from the storage of combustible materials and from the paraffin dispenser(s)? [ ]
64. Are knives stored in original containers or by some other means to avoid injury in handling and storage? [ ]
65. With regard to all specimens containing body fluids, are there written procedures for:
    Transport and handling of specimens? [ ]
    Labeled, well-constructed containers? [ ]
    Secure lids to prevent leakage? [ ]
66. Are infectious tissues and other contaminated materials disposed of to minimize any danger to professional, technical, and custodial workers? [ ]
67. Is there a written procedure for disposal of infectious specimens and contaminated materials such as those found in the cytology specimen areas? [ ]
68. Is there a written procedure for the special handling of highly infectious materials? [ ]
69. Are formaldehyde and xylene fume concentrations maintained at a permissible limit? [ ]
70. Are safety policies and procedures written and implemented for electron microscopy sample preparations and instrument operations? [ ]
71. Is a safety hood available for use with osmium tetroxide and other volatile or hazardous materials? [ ]

72. Are there written policies and procedures for handling and disposal of osmium tetroxide and other highly hazardous chemicals used in the electron microscopy laboratory?   [ ]
73. Has the electron microscope been checked for x-ray leakage at the time of installation and after major repairs? (Periodic monitoring is also required for devices operating at 70,000 volts or by above.)   [ ]
74. Is there a defined program to reduce the amount of hazardous waste generated by the entire laboratory?   [ ]
        Recycling?   [ ]
        Eliminations?   [ ]
        Substitution?   [ ]
        Conservation?   [ ]

A2 RESOURCE MATERIAL

A2.1 OSHA AND OTHER PUBLICATIONS

Single free copies of the following publications may be obtained from OSHA field offices or writing to the OSHA Publications Office, 200 Constitution Ave NW, Room N3101, Washington, DC 20210.

A2.1.1 PAMPHLETS

OSHA-2056	All About OSHA
OSHA-2098	OSHA Inspections
OSHA-3021	OSHA: Employee Workplace Rights
OSHA-3084	Chemical Hazard Communication
OSHA-3047	Consultation Services for the Employer
OSHA-3088	How to Prepare for Workplace Emergencies
OSHA-3071	Job Hazard Analysis
OSHA-3077	Personal Protective Equipment
OSHA-3079	Respiratory Protection
OSHA-3085	OSHA Computerized Information System (contains chemical information file of sampling and analytical methods of analysis for more than 750 workplace chemicals)
OSHA-3112	Air Contaminants: Permissible Limits
OSHA-3111	Hazard Communication Guidelines for Compliance
OSHA-3071	Job Hazard Analysis
OSHA-2254	Training Requirements in OSHA Standards and Training Guidelines
OSHA-3119	Exposure to Hazardous Chemicals in Laboratories
OSHA-200	Record Keeping Requirements for Occupational Injury and Illness

A2.1.2 FACT SHEETS

Fact Sheet No. OSHA 89-15	State Job Safety and Health Programs
Fact Sheet No. OSHA 86-08	Protect Yourself with Personal Protective Equipment
Fact Sheet No. OSHA 89-32	Control of Hazardous Energy Sources (Lock-out/Tag-out)
Fact Sheet No. OSHA 87-02	Inspecting for Job Safety and Health Hazards
Fact Sheet No. OSHA 90-33	Occupational Exposure to Hazardous Chemicals in Laboratories
Fact Sheet No. OSHA 91-44	OSHA Emergency Hot-line
Fact Sheet No. OSHA 92-46	Bloodborne Pathogens Final Standard: Summary of Key Provisions

Bloodborne Facts   Hepatitis B Vaccination: Protection for You
                                    Protect Yourself When Handling Sharps
                                    Reporting Exposure Incidents
                                    Personal Protective Equipment Cuts Risks
                                    Holding the Line on Contamination

A2.1.3 OSHA STANDARDS

OSHA 29 CFR 1910	Hazardous Waste Operations and Emergency Response; Final Rule, April 13, 1990
OSHA 29 CFR 1910.1030	Occupational Exposure to Bloodborne Pathogens; Final Rule, December 6, 1991
OSHA 29 CFR 1910.1450	Occupational Exposures to Hazardous Chemicals in Laboratories; Final Rule, January 31, 1990
OSHA 29 CFR 1910.1048	Occupational Exposure to Formaldehyde, December 5, 1987; Final Rule, May 27, 1992
OSHA 29 CFR 1910.1028	Benzene
OSHA 29 CFR 1910.1001-1016	Specified Carcinogens
OSHA 29 CFR 1910.1200	Hazard Communication Standard, May 23, 1988

Also OSHA enforcement procedures (specific documents for each of the above standards), Office of Health Compliance Assistance (OSHA Instruction CPL documents).

A2.1.4 ADDITIONAL TRAINING RESOURCES

American Chemical Society, Room 502, 1155 Sixteenth Street, Washington, DC 20036. *Chemical and Engineering News* (about 12 pages, free subscription), Waste Management Manual for Laboratory Personnel (free single copies).

American Society of Clinical Pathologists, PO Box 98346, Chicago, IL 60693-8346 (800) 621-4142. OSHA's Bloodborne Pathogens Standard: Compliance in the Clinical Laboratory (video, monograph, and pre/post tests).

Becton-Dickinson and Company, 1 Becton Drive, Franklin Lakes, NJ 07417 (201) 847-7446. For Your Protection: The OSHA Regulations on Bloodborne Pathogens (OSHA training program developed with the American Medical Association). Also, Becton-Dickinson Safety Compliance Initiative Program (focus on needle stick prevention developed with the National League of Nursing).

Center for Accelerated Learning, 1103 Wisconsin Street, Lake Geneva, WI 53147 (414) 248-7070. Education and training classes on OSHA regulations.

Centers for Disease Control and Prevention, Clearinghouse, Box 6003, Rockville, MD 20849-6003. *AIDS and HIV Surveillance Report*. Also other publications for laboratory applications.

Chemical Safety Associates, 9163 Chesapeake Drive, San Diego, CA 92123 (619) 647-8970. A Model Exposure Control Plan (for bloodborne pathogens).

Edge Technologies, 610 River Street, Hoboken, NJ 07030 (201) 798-1893. Biosafety Training for Laboratory Employees and Chemical Safety in the Laboratory (both computer-based training programs).

Environmental Protection Agency, Environmental Assistance Division TS-799, Office of Toxic Substances, 401 M Street SW, Washington, DC 20460. *Chemicals in Progress* (about 28 pages, six issues per year, by subscription).

Genium Publishing Corporation, Department EPGOA, Room 225, 1145 Catalyn Street, Schenectady, NY 12303-1836 (518) 377-8854. *Right-to-Know Pocket Guide for Laboratory Employees* (88-page pamphlet on essential OSHA requirements, free single copies).

Guidance Associates, The Center for Humanities, PO Box 1000, Mount Kisco, NY 10549-0010 (800) 431-1242. AIDS Prevention for Laboratory Professionals and AIDS Prevention for Support Service Employees (both developed in conjunction with College of American Pathologists).

Kimberly-Clark Corporation, Roswell, GA. OSHA regulation helpline: (800) 524-3511.

National Committee for Clinical Laboratory Standards, 771 E Lancaster, Villanova, PA 19085 (215) 527-8390. Laboratory Document Set SC10 Protection of Laboratory Workers from Infectious Disease (M29).

National Institute of Environmental Health Services, National Toxicology Program Public Information Office, Box 12233, Research Triangle Park, NC 27709 (919) 541-3991. Technical report series—a number of chemical investigations available.

National Institute for Occupational Safety and Health, Nordic Expert Group for Documentation of Occupational Exposure Limits, Publications Dissemination, DSDTT, 4676 Columbia Parkway, Cincinnati, OH 45226. Basis for an Occupational Health Standard: Ethyl Ether (publication #93-103). Also numerous publications for laboratory applications (chlorofluorocarbon #113, spray coolants).

National Laboratory Training Network, South Central Area, 325 Loyola, 7th Floor, New Orleans, LA 70112.

OSHA Training Institute, 1555 Times Drive, Des Plaines, IL 60018 (312) 297-4810. Consultation and training classes on OSHA regulations.

Savant Audiovisuals Inc, 801 E Chapman Avenue, Fullerton, CA 92634 (800) 472-8268. Guide to OSHA's Bloodborne Pathogen Standard and others regarding OSHA standards.

Syntex Public Affairs Department, 340 Hillview Avenue, Palo Alto, CA 94303 (301) 210-6781. Universal Precautions in the Laboratory, Universal Precautions for Health Care Workers, and Universal Precautions for Health Care Professions. Films are free.

Target Training Technologies, Formula for Safety, 340 Hungerford Drive, Rockville, MD 20850. Planning for Safety in Laboratories, Hood and Glove Boxes, Glassware, Eye Protection, Basic Chemical Hazards, Spills in the Laboratory, Waste Disposal, Laboratory Housekeeping, Laboratory Gloves (10- to 12-minute safety videos).

A2.2 OSHA AND STATE CONSULTATION SERVICES

Consultation programs funded by OSHA and delivered by well-trained professional staff members of state governments are provided free to employers who request help. Whether identifying and correcting specific hazards, improving health and safety programs, and/or providing further assistance in training and education, these services provide comprehensive consultation, which includes an appraisal of all workplace hazards, practices, and job health and safety programs. Conferences and agreements with employers, assistance in implementation of recommendations and a follow-up appraisal to ensure that any required correction is made is also provided. For more information on this program, contact your appropriate state office.

Alabama	On Site Construction Project (205) 348-3033
Alaska	Department of Labor Occupational Safety and Health (907) 264-2599
Arizona	Consultation and Training, Division of Occupational Health and Safety (602) 255-5795
Arkansas	OSHA Consultation, Department of Labor (501) 682-4522
California	Department of Industrial Relations (415) 557-2870

Colorado	Occupation Health and Safety Section, Institute of Rural Environmental Health (303)491-6151
Connecticut	Division of Occupational Safety and Health, Department of Labor (203) 566-4550
Delaware	Occupational Safety and Health, Division of Industrial Affairs (302) 571-3908
District of Columbia	Occupational Safety and Health, DC Department of Employment Services (202) 576-6339
Florida	Onsite Construction Program, Bureau of Safety and Health (904) 488-3044
Georgia	Onsite Construction Program, Georgia-Tech Research Institute (404) 894-3806
Guam	Onsite Construction, International Trade Center (671) 646-9246
Hawaii	Division of Occupational Safety and Health (808) 548-7510
Idaho	Safety and Health Consultation (208) 385- 3283
Illinois	Division of Industrial Affairs (312) 917- 2339
Indiana	Bureau of Safety, Education and Training (317) 232-2688
Iowa	Consultation Program, Division of Labor (515) 281-5352
Kansas	Consultation Program, Department of Human Resources (913) 296-4386
Kentucky	Consultation and Training, OSHA Program, Labor Cabinet (502) 564-6895
Louisiana	Consultation Program, Department of Labor (504) 925-6005
Maine	Division of Industrial Safety, Division of Labor and Industry (301) 333-4218
Massachusetts	Consultation Program, Division of Industrial Safety (617) 727-3567
Michigan	Special Programs Sections, Department of Public Health (517) 335-8250
Minnesota	Consultation Division (Safety), Department of Labor and Industry (612) 623-5510
Mississippi	Onsite Consultation Program, Division Occupational Safety and Health (601) 965-4606
Missouri	Onsite Construction Program, Division of Labor Standards (314) 751-3403
Montana	Bureau of Safety and Health, Division of Worker's Compensation (406) 444-6418
Nebraska	Division of Safety, Labor and Safety, Department of Labor (402) 471- 4717
Nevada	Training and Consultation, Division of Occupational Safety and Health (702) 789-0546
New Hampshire	Onsite Construction Program, Department of Labor (603) 271-3170
New Jersey	Division of Workplace Standards, Department of Labor (609) 984-3507
New Mexico	OSHA Consultation Service, Bureau of Heath and Safety (505) 827-2885
New York	Division of Health and Safety, Department of Labor (718) 797-7648
North Carolina	Consultative Services, Department of Labor (919) 733-2360
North Dakota	Environmental Engineering, Department of Health (701) 224-2348
Ohio	Onsite Construction, Department of Industrial Relations (614) 644-2631
Oklahoma	OSHA Division, Department of Labor (405) 235-0530 x240
Oregon	Consultation Program, Employer Services (503) 378-2890
Pennsylvania	Indiana University of Pennsylvania, Safety Sciences Department (412) 357-2561
Puerto Rico	Occupation Safety and Health, Department of Labor (809) 745-2134
Rhode Island	Occupational Health, Department of Health (401) 277-2438
South Carolina	Onsite Construction Program (803) 734-9599
Tennessee	OSHA Consultive Services, Department of Labor (615) 741-2793
Texas	Occupational Health and Safety, Department of Health (512) 458-7287
Utah	Safety and Health Consultation Service (801) 530-6868
Vermont	Division of Occupational Safety and Health, Department of Labor (802) 828-2765
Virginia	Department of Labor and Industry (804) 367-1986
Virgin Islands	Occupational Safety and Health, Department of Labor (809) 772-1315
Washington	Voluntary Services, Department of Labor and Industry (206) 586-0961
West Virginia	Department of Labor (304) 348-7890
Wisconsin	Occupational Health, Department of Health and Social Services (608) 266-8579

Wyoming   Occupational Health and Safety (307) 777-7786
Other Important
   Resources Consultation Training Coordination: OSHA Training Institute,
              1555 Times Drive, Des Plaines, IL 60018 (708) 297-4810
              Laboratory Services Agreement: Wisconsin Occupational Health Laboratory,
              979 Jonathan Drive, Madison, WI 53713 (608) 263-8807

A2.3 IMPORTANT TELEPHONE NUMBERS

American Board of Industrial Hygienists ....(517) 321-2638
American Chemical Society (ACS) ....(800) 227-5558
American Conference of Governmental Industrial Hygienists ....(513) 661-7881
American Industrial Hygiene Association ....(216) 873-2442
American Industrial Hygiene Institute (ANSI) ....(212) 642-4900
American Society of Safety Engineers ....(708) 692-4121
American Society for Testing Materials (ASTM) ....(215) 299-5400
College of American Pathologists (CAP) Spill Hot-line ....(800) 443-3544
Centers for Disease Control and Prevention (CDC) ....(404) 639-3535
Chemical Abstracts Service, American Chemical Society ....(614) 447-3698
Chemical Health and Safety Division, American Chemical Society ....(202) 872-4600
Chemical Manufacturers Association (CMA) ....(202) 887-1100
Chemical Referral Hot-line (CMA) ....(800) 262-8200
ChemTrec (provides information in event of hazardous spill) ....(800) 424-9300
Environmental Document Service ....(800) 424-9068
Environmental Hazardous Management Institute ....(603) 868-1496
Environmental Protection Agency Small Business Hotline ....(800) 368-5888
Food and Drug Administration (FDA) ....(301) 443-1544
Food and Drug Administration (FDA) Problem Reporting Program ....(800) 638-6725
Formaldehyde Institute ....(202) 659-0060
Government Printing Office for Publications ....(202) 512-2457
Joint Commission on Accreditation of Hospitals (JCOAH) ....(708) 916-3600
National Audio-Visual Center ....(301) 763-1896
National Fire Protection Agency (NFPA) ....(617) 770-3000
National Institute of Occupational Safety and Health (NIOSH) ....(513) 533-8236
NIOSH Information Line ....(800) 356-4674
National Response Center (when fire, explosion, or release occurs) ....(800) 424-8802
National Society for Histotechnology (anatomic pathology) ....(301) 262-6221
OSHA Central Information Line ....(800) 321-6742
Poison Control Center ....(800) 535-0525
RCRA/Superfund Hot-line ....(800) 424-9346
Substance Identification Information ....(800) 848-6538
Safety Equipment Institute ....(703) 525-1695
Underwriters Laboratories (UL) ....(708) 272-1695
US Department of Health and Human Resources ....(202) 619-0257
US Department of Transportation (DOT) ....(202) 366-4000
US Public Health Service ....(301) 443-2403

ACCL	American Conference on Chemical Labeling
ACGIH	American Conference of Governmental Industrial Hygienist, 6500 Glenway Avenue, Building D-7, Cincinnati, OH 45211-4438 (513) 661-7881
ACH	Air changes per hour—movement of a specific volume of air in a given period of time
ACS	American Chemical Society (800) 227-5558
Action Level	Level of exposure at which OSHA regulations for protective programs must be put into effect
Acute	An adverse effect on the human body with symptoms of high severity coming quickly into crisis. Acute effects are usually the result of short-term exposures.
Acute toxicity	The ability of a substance to cause poisonous effects resulting in severe biological harm or death after a single exposure or dose
Accumulation of waste	EPA has set restrictions on how much waste may be accumulated on-site.
ADI	Acceptable daily intake
Adsorb	Adherence of gases, solutes, or liquids in an extremely thin layer of molecules to the surfaces of solid bodies or liquids with which they are in contact
AEA	Atomic Energy Act
AICE	American Institute of Chemical Engineers
AIHC	American Industrial Health Council
AL	Acceptable level
ALARA	As low as reasonably achievable
ALK	Alkali
ALR	Allergenic effects
Ambient	An encompassing atmosphere
American Industrial Hygiene Association	345 White Pond Drive, Akron, OH 44320 (216) 873-2442
American Society of Safety Engineers	1800 E Oakton Street, Philadelphia, PA 19103 (215) 299-5400
Anhydride	Compound derived from another such as an acid, by removal of water elements
Anhydrous	Free from water and especially water crystallization
Annual Report on	List of substances that either are known or anticipated to be carcinogens. Published by the
Carcinogens	National Toxicology Program (NTP), available from the National Technical Information Service (NTIS), US Department of Commerce, 5285 Port Royal Road, Springfield, PA 22161 (703) 487-4600
ANSI	American National Standards Institute, 1014 Broadway, New York, NY 10018 (212) 642-4900; formulates guidelines for precautionary labeling; private organization that works with the ACS and the ACCL
AO	Area office
Apnea	Transient cessation of respiration
"APPROVED"	As stated in OSHA standards, this means (unless otherwise indicated) approved or listed by at least one of the following nationally recognized testing laboratories: Underwriters Laboratories Inc and Factory Mutual Research; beware of "approved" claims that may be made regarding certain products; be sure you understand whose approval is indicated and if it is actually relevant to the product
APT	Associated Pharmacists and Toxicologists
Argyria	Poisoning by silver or its compounds

ASHRAE	American Society of Heating, Refrigeration, and Air Conditioning Engineers Inc
ASTM	American Society for Testing and Materials; develops voluntary standards for materials, products, systems, and services.
Asphyxiant	Chemical that replaces oxygen in the air and can cause death by suffocation such as nitrogen, carbon dioxide, and hydrogen sulfide
Ataxia	Inability to coordinate voluntary muscular movements, which is symptomatic of some neurological disorders
ATERIS	Air Toxics Exposure and Risk Information System (ORD)
ATSDR	Agency for Toxic Substances and Disease Registry (HHS)
Autoignition temperature	The minimum temperature at which a substance will ignite into fire without a flame or spark
Base	Compound that yields hydroxyl ions in aqueous solutions, and which reacts with acids to form water and a salt
Bioconcentrative	Substances that living organisms extract and accumulate to levels greater than those in the surrounding environment, which may be harmful when so accumulated
"Biodegradable"	Not automatically safe to dispose of down the drain; certain chemicals like formaldehyde, xylene, or toluene are biodegradable (over a period of time or may kill treatment plant bacteria).
BLD	Blood effects
Bleach, household	Hypochlorite; accepted in a 1:10 solution as an effective decontaminant for potentially infectious surfaces
Blood	Human blood, human components, and products made from human blood
Bloodborne pathogen	Pathogenic microorganisms that are present in human blood and can cause disease in humans, including, but are not limited to, hepatitis B virus (HBV) and human immunodeficiency virus (HIV)
BLS	Bureau of Labor Statistics
BOM	Bureau of Mines
BTU	British thermal unit
Bonding	Provision of metal-to-metal contact (usually by wire) between two containers to prevent generation of static electrical sparks
"C" (ceiling)	The maximum allowable exposure limit for an airborne substance, not to be exceeded even momentarily (see TLV)
CAA	Clean Air Act (1990)—requires EPA to develop rules for laboratory emissions
CAER	Community awareness and emergency response
CAFO	Consent agreement final order
CAG	Carcinogenic assessment group
CAMP	Continuous air monitoring program
CAP	College of American Pathologists, 325 Waukegan Road, Northfield, IL 60093-2750 (800) 323-4040
CAR, CARC	Carcinogen—substance capable of causing cancer
CAS	Chemical Abstracts Service, PO Box 3012, Columbus, OH 43210 (614) 421-6940
CAS No.	A registry number that has been assigned to the chemical by the CAS, which identifies the chemicals and any pseudonyms
Caustic	Capable of destroying or eating away by chemical action; corrosive
CCBW	Chemically contaminated biological waste
CCID	Confidential chemical identification system
CDC	Centers for Disease Control and Prevention, 1600 Clifton Road NE, Atlanta, GA 30333 (404) 639-3535

CEO	Chief Executive Officer
CEPP	Chemical emergency preparedness plan
CERCLA	Comprehensive Environmental Response, Compensation, and Liability Act (1980); authorizes EPA to clean up hazardous waste (see Superfund Amendment).
CEL	Ceiling exposure limit; concentrations that should never be exceeded
CFM	cubic feet per minute
CFR	Code of Federal Regulations—the collection of rules and regulations originally published in the Federal Register by various government departments and agencies. OSHA regulations are found in the 29 CFR, EPA regulations in the 40 CFR, and the Department of Transportation regulations in the 49 CFR.
CFS	cubic feet per second
Chemical Hygiene Officer	Employee designated by the employer, who is qualified by training or experience to provide technical guidance in the development and implementation of the provisions of the Chemical Hygiene Plan
Chemical Hygiene Plan	Written program developed and implemented by the employer that sets forth procedures, equipment, personal protective equipment, and work practices that are capable of protecting employees from the health hazards of chemicals used in the workplace
Chemical Referral Center Hot-line	(800) 262-8200
Chemical agent	A wide variety of agents (usually fluids) that have a high potential for body entry by various means; some are more toxic than others and require special measures of control for safety and environmental reasons.
Chemical name	Name designated by the International Union of Pure and Applied Chemistry, Chemical Abstracts Service, or a name that clearly identifies the chemical for hazard-evaluation purposes
ChemTrek	Chemical Transportation Emergency Center; national center that provides emergency information about specific chemicals on request (800) 424-9300
CHIP	Chemical Hazard Information Profile (Toxic Substance Control Act)
Chronic	An adverse effect on the human body with symptoms that develop slowly over a long period of time or frequently recur
Chronic effect	An adverse effect on humans or animals with symptoms that develop slowly over a long period of time or which recur frequently
Chronic toxicity	Adverse effects that result from multiple doses of a chemical or from multiple exposures; usually used to describe effects in experimental animals
CMA	Chemical Manufacturers Association, 2501 M Street NW, Washington, DC 20037-1303 (202) 887-1100
COC	Cleveland Open Cup; method for testing flash point
Combustible	A material that is able to catch fire and burn
Combustible liquid	Any liquid having a flash point at or above 100°F, but below 200°F
Community	Known as SARA Title III; passed by Congress as individual states and communities began to
Right-to-Know Law	legislate the issue of the right to know
Contaminated	The presence or the reasonably anticipated presence of blood or other potentially infectious materials on an item or surface
Contaminated sharps	Any contaminated object that can penetrate the skin including needles, scalpels, broken glass, broken capillary tubes, and exposed ends of dental wires
Contaminated laundry	Laundry that has been soiled with blood or other potentially infectious materials or may contain sharps

COR	Corrosive—a chemical that causes visible destruction or irreversible damage to living tissue
CPC	Chemical protective clothing
CPF	Carcinogenic potency factor
CPSC	Consumer Product Safety Commission
CSIN	Chemical Substances Information Network
CTARC	Chemical Testing and Assessment Research Commission
Cum	Cumulative effects
CWA	Clean Water Act (1986), Water Quality Act (1987)—Restores and maintains the physical, chemical, and biological integrity of the nation's waterways and controls nonpoint source emissions.
CWTC	Chemical Waste Transportation Council
Decontamination	Procedure used to eliminate or reduce microbial concentration to a safe level with respect to the transmission of infection. Decontamination is often accomplished by using sterilization and disinfection procedures.
Degradation	The destructive effect of a chemical on a piece of chemical-protective clothing, by partially dissolving, softening, hardening, or completely destroying
Deliquescent	Tending to melt or dissolve, especially tending to undergo gradual dissolution and liquefaction by the attraction and absorption of moisture from air
Designated area	An area that may be used for work with "select carcinogens," reproductive toxins, or substances that have a high degree of acute toxicity
Disinfection	Procedure that kills pathogenic microorganisms but not necessarily their spores; chemical germicides used as disinfectants should only be used on inanimate surfaces and never on skin or body tissues.
Disposal regulations	OSHA does not regulate or have any disposal regulations; the EPA regulates what is considered hazardous waste
DOC	Department of Commerce
DOE	Department of Energy
Dosimeter	Instrument that measures exposure to radiation
DOT	Department of Transportation, 400 7th Street SW, Washington DC 20590 (202) 366-4000
Dyspnea	Difficult or labored respiration
EENET	Emergency Education Network (FEMA)
EHS	Extremely hazardous substance
ELI	Environmental Law Institute
Emergency Response Guidebook	Published by the Department of Transportation for initial response to hazardous materials–related incidents
Engineering controls	Controls (eg, sharps disposal containers, self-sheathing needles, etc) that isolate or remove the bloodborne pathogens hazard from the workplace
Environmental Hazardous Management Institute	Box 932, Durham, NH 03824 (603) 868-1496
EPA	Environmental Protection Agency, Public Affairs, 401 M Street NW, Washington, DC 20460 (202) 260-2090
EPA Hazardous Waste No.	Number assigned by the EPA to each hazardous waste type
EPA Identification No.	Number assigned by the EPA to each generator, transporter, and treatment, storage, or disposal facility

Epidemiology	Study of diseases and epidemics, comparing who contracts a disease with other factors such as occupation, age, or sex, identification of patterns, and potential causes of the disease
ERT	Emergency response team
Explosive	Material that produces sudden, almost instantaneous release of energy in the form of pressure, gas, and heat when subjected to sudden shock, pressure, or high temperature
Exposure Incident	Specific eye, mouth, other mucous membrane, nonintact skin, or parenteral contact with blood or other potentially infectious materials that results from the performance of an employee's duties
FDA	Food and Drug Administration, General Information, 5600 Fishers Lane, Rockville, MD 20857 (301) 443-1544
FDA Problem Reporting Program	(800) 638-6725
Flammable	Substance which ignites easily and burns rapidly
Flammable Limits in Air	The range of gas or vapor concentrations that will burn or explode if ignition source is present
FLP	Flash point—minimum temperature at which there is enough vapor to ignite in air when a source of ignition is present
FR	Federal Register
FMR	Factory Mutual Research; recognized independent testing laboratory established by the insurance industry to which manufacturers submit their products for evaluation of ability to meet safety requirements
Fusible Link Device	Strip that melts at 160°F and is used to hold spring-loaded covers of tanks and doors of storage cabinets; in case of fire, or any other source of extreme heat, the cover or door closes to protect contents
General exhaust	Method for ventilating air with contaminants from a general work area
Generator	A facility that generates a minimum monthly quantity of hazardous waste as defined by regulations. The Medical Waste Tracking Act defines a generator by occupation or activity rather than by quantity of waste generated. Generators of medical waste include health care providers, veterinarians, research laboratories, or facilities involved in treating, diagnosing, or immunizing humans (see also small and large quantity generators).
Government Printing Office	To order publications, Washington, DC 20402-9371 (202) 512-2457
GRAS	Generally regarded as safe—an FDA designation for descriptions used only for foods, not for chemical use
Grounding	Provision of contact between container and "ground" (usually by wire) to prevent generation of static electric sparks
Handwashing facilities	A facility providing an adequate supply of running potable water, soap, and single use towels or hot air drying machine
Hazardous chemical	Any chemical for which there is significant evidence that it is a physical or health hazard
Hazardous material	Material designated to be capable of posing an unreasonable risk to health, safety, or property when transported
Hazardous waste	Any substance that singly, or in combination, poses an immediate or potential threat to human health or to the environment and which singly, or in combination, requires special handling, processing, or disposal because it is flammable, explosive, reactive, corrosive, toxic, carcinogenic, infectious, bioconcentrative, potentially lethal, irritating, or strongly sensitizing

HBV	Hepatitis B virus
HC	Hydrocarbon—a chemical compound consisting entirely of carbon and hydrogen
Health hazard (chemical)	Chemical that has an acute or chronic health effect, such as carcinogens, toxicins, irritants, corrosives, and sensitizers
HEPA	High-efficiency particulate air filter
Hepatoxin	A chemical that can produce liver damage in man such as carbon tetrachloride and nitrosamines
HIV	Human immunodeficiency virus
HMIS	Hazardous Material Identification System—labeling system that uses letters, numbers, and symbols to communicate hazard information
HMTA	Hazardous Materials Transportation Act
Hood capture efficiency	The emissions from a process that are captured by hood and directed into the control device, expressed as a percent of all emissions
HRSA	Health Resources and Services Administration (Federal)
HVAC	Heating, ventilation, and air conditioning (systems)
Hypergolic	Igniting upon contact of components without external aid such as a spark
IARC	International Agency for Research on Cancer; IARC publications, WHO Publications Center, 49 Sheridan Street, Albany, NY 12210; information on human carcinogens
IAQ	Indoor air quality
ICWM	Institute for Chemical Waste Management
IDLH	Immediately dangerous to life or health; maximum concentration that an individual could survive within 30 minutes without symptoms or irreversible health effects
Ignitable	A substance that, under standard temperature and pressure, is capable of causing fire through friction, absorption of moisture, or other spontaneous chemical change and, when ignited, will burn vigorously and persistently
Incompatability	Materials, substances, and conditions to avoid to prevent hazardous reactions that may result (of chemicals) in toxic vapors and/or reactions resulting in explosion or fire
Infectious Agents	Sources that cause infections by inhalation, ingestion, or direct contact with the host material
Infectious Waste	Waste containing, or potentially containing, pathogens of sufficient virulence and quantity that exposure to it by a susceptible host could result in the development by the host of a communicable disease
Ingestion	Means of taking chemicals or other substances into the body by swallowing
Inhalation	Breathing chemicals or other substances into the body through the lungs
Inhibitor	A chemical that is added to another substance to keep an undesirable chemical reaction from occurring
"In Vitro Diagnostic Use"	Histology chemical labeling suitable for processing and staining, established by the FDA; "for laboratory use only" and "for institutional use only" are terms used that are not in compliance with the FDA
IRR	Irritant—a substance that can cause irritation of skin, eyes, or respiratory tract; effects may be acute from a single high-level exposure or chronic from repeated low-level exposures such as chlorine, nitrogen dioxide, and nitric acid.
IUPAC	International Union of Pure and Applied Chemistry
JCOAH	Joint Commission on Accreditation of Hospitals, 1 Renaissance Boulevard, Oakbrook Terrace, IL 60181
Lab Pack	An overpacked container (such as a drum) containing small tightly sealed containers of hazardous waste with an absorbent material filling the voids in the outer container (drum)

Laboratory	A facility in which the "laboratory use of hazardous chemicals" occurs; a workplace where relatively small quantities of hazardous chemicals are used on a nonproduction basis
Laboratory scale	Work with substances in which the containers used for reactions, transfers, and other handling of substances are designed to be easily and safely manipulated by one person; "laboratory scale" excludes those workplaces whose function is to produce commercial quantities of materials.
Laboratory use of chemical	Handling or use of such chemicals in which all of the following conditions are met: hazardous chemicals manipulations are carried out on a "laboratory scale"; multiple chemical procedures or chemicals are used; procedures involved are not part of a production process; and protective laboratory practices and equipment are available and in common use to minimize the potential for employee exposure to hazardous chemicals.
Large Quantity Generator	A generator who produces 1000 kg or more of hazardous waste in any calendar month
LD50	The dose that causes death in 50% of the animals exposed by swallowing a substance; a measure of acute toxicity
LEL	Lower explosive limit
LFL	Lower flammability limit
LOAEL	Lowest observed adverse effect level
LOC	Level of concern
LOEL	Lowest observed effect level
Manifest	A document that identifies the type of waste, generator, transporter, and the method and site of disposal. It is required by regulatory authorities when shipping hazardous waste materials.
MATC	Maximum allowable toxicant concentration
MCL	Maximum contaminant level
Medical consultation	Consultation that takes place between an employee and a licensed physician for the purpose of determining what medical examinations or procedures, if any, are appropriate in cases in which a significant exposure to a hazardous chemical may have taken place
Medical Waste Tracking Act	Authorizes the EPA to promulgate and define and track medical waste.
Miscible	The extent to which liquids or gases can be blended
Monitoring, initial	Employee monitoring required for any substance regulated by a standard if there is reason to believe that exposure levels for that substance routinely exceed the action level
Monitoring, periodic	Prescribed mandatory monitoring when employee exposures have exceeded the action level or permissible exposure limit
MMWR	Morbidity and Mortality Weekly Report; published by CDC summarizing current epidemiological data
MSDS	Material Safety Data Sheet
MSHA	Mine Safety and Health Administration
Mucous membrane	The protective lining of cells in the mouth, throat, and throughout the respiratory and digestive system
Mutagen	A substance capable of changing cells in such a way that future cell generations are affected; mutagenic substances are usually considered suspect carcinogens
NA, N/A	Not applicable; not available
NBS	National Bureau of Standards

NCCLS	National Committee for Clinical Laboratory Standards, 771 East Lancaster Avenue, Villanova, PA 19085
Nephrotoxin	Chemical that produces kidney damage, such as uranium and the halogenated hydrocarbons that are commonly found in many solvents
NETC	National Emergency Training Center
Neurotoxin	Chemical that has toxic effects on the nervous system, such as mercury and carbon disulfide
NFPA	National Fire Protection Agency, Batterymarch Park, Quincy, Massachusetts (617) 770-3000
NFPA Code 30	Code developed by the NFPA to cover safe storage and handling of flammable and combustible liquids
NIH	National Institutes of Health
NIMBY	Not in my backyard
NOAEL	No observed adverse effect level
NIOSH	National Institute of Occupational Safety and Health; Superintendent of Documents, US Government Printing Office, Washington, DC 20402 (800) 356-4674
"Nontoxic"	OSHA and the EPA have separate definitions of toxicity; understand which definition is being referred to when making such a decision regarding a chemical
nos	Not Otherwise Specified; often used in DOT classifications and regulations
NRC	Nuclear Regulatory Commission; regulates radioactive waste
NRC	National Research Council, the operating arm of the National Academy of Sciences and the National Academy of Engineering
NRC	National Response Center; notification center that must be informed of any significant oil or chemical spills or incidents that could affect the environment (800) 424-8802
NSH	National Society for Histotechnology
NTE	Not to exceed
NTP	National Toxicology Program, annual report on carcinogens
Occupational Exposure	Reasonably anticipated skin, eye, mucous membrane, or parenteral contact with blood or other potentially infectious materials that may result from the performance of an employee's duties
Oncogenic	Substance that causes tumors, both benign and malignant
OPIM	Other potentially infectious material: (1) the following human body fluids: semen, vaginal secretions, cerebrospinal fluid, synovial fluid, pleural fluid, pericardial fluid, peritoneal fluid, amniotic fluid, saliva in dental procedures, any body fluid that is visibly contaminated with blood and all body fluids in situations where it is difficult or impossible to differentiate between body fluids; (2) any unfixed tissue or organ (other than intact skin) from a human (living or dead); (3) HIV-containing cell or tissue cultures, organ cultures, and HIV or HBV-containing culture medium or other solutions and blood, organs, or other tissues from experimental animals infected with HIV or HBV
Organic peroxide	An organic compound that contains the bivalent -0-0- structure and is considered to be a structural derivative of hydrogen peroxide where one or both of the hydrogen atoms have been replaced by an organic radical
ORM	Other regulated material
OSHA	Occupational Safety and Health Administration, 200 Constitution Avenue, Washington, DC 20210 (202) 523-6091; regulatory branch of the Department of Labor concerned with employee safety and health

OSHA Publications	Room N-3101, 200 Constitution Ave, NW, Washington, DC 20210 (202) 523-9667
OSHA Information and Consumer Affairs	Room N-3649, 200 Constitution Ave, NW, Washington, DC 20210 (202) 523-8151
Oxidizer	Substance/chemical that yields oxygen readily to stimulate the combustion of organic matter
Oxy	Oxidizer
Parenteral	Exposure occurring as the result of piercing the skin barrier (eg, subcutaneous, intramuscular, intravenous routes)
PCB	Polychlorinated biphenyl; EPA interprets this term to include monochlorobiphenyls.
PCP	Pneumocystis carinii pneumonia; the organism does not cause disease among persons with a normal immune system.
PEL	Permissible Exposure Limit; the legally allowed concentration in the workplace that is considered a safe level of exposure for an 8-hour, 40 hour-per-week workshift
Percent volatile by volume	Indicates how much of a substance will evaporate or vaporize at 70°F; a substance like gasoline is 100% volatile, indicating that it will vaporize entirely over a period of time
pH	A measure of how acidic or caustic (basic) a substance is on a scale of 1 to 14; a pH of 1 indicates that a substance is very acidic; and a pH of 14 indicates that a substance is very caustic (basic).
Physical agent	Workplace sources recognized for their potential effects on the body; heat exposure or excessive noise levels are examples of this risk group.
Physical hazard	A chemical with significant evidence that it is a combustible liquid, a compressed gas, explosive, flammable, an organic peroxide, an oxidizer, pyrophoric, unstable (reactive), or water-reactive
PHS	Public Health Service
PIM	Potentially infectious material
PMR	Proportioned mortality ratio
POE	Point of exposure
POHC	Principal organic hazardous constituent; an organic chemical constituent identified by the EPA that is to be burned in an incinerator
Poison, Class A	Extremely dangerous poisonous gases that can kill in very small quantities such as phosgene and hydrocyanic acid (DOT)
Poison, Class B	A solid or liquid substance that is toxic to humans (DOT)
Polymerization	A reaction in which small molecules combine to form larger molecules; when hazardous polymerization occurs it is an uncontrolled chemical reaction that releases great amounts of energy.
POTW	Publicly Owned Treatment Works
PPC	Personal protective clothing
PPE	Personal protective equipment
PR (respirator)	A disposable particulate respirator (respiratory protective device (face mask) that is designed to filter out particles 1 to 5 microns in diameter
Pressure Relief	A device or system to release vapor at a safe pressure to prevent pressure buildup and rupture of a closed container; the spout cap of a safety can is such a device.
ppm	parts per million; how many parts of a substance exist in a million parts of air
psi	pounds per square inch; unit for measuring pressure
Pyrophoric	Chemical capable of self-igniting when exposed to air
RCRA	Resource Conservation and Recovery Act (1976); amended by the EPA in 1980; established a cradle-to-grave system for management of hazardous waste (Hazardous Solid Waste Amendment)

Reactive substance	Any material that combines violently with water, air, or other chemicals to generate heat, (unstable) pressure, or toxic fumes (eg, bleach combined with ammonia releases noxious fumes)
Reducing agent	Chemical that combines with oxygen or loses electrons to a reaction
Reproductive toxins	Chemicals that affect the reproductive capabilities producing chromosomal damage (mutagens) and effects on fetuses (teratogenesis)
REL	Recommended exposure limit—highest allowable airborne concentration of a substance that is not anticipated to create health hazards; may be expressed as CEL or TWA.
Regulated waste	Liquid or semiliquid blood or other potentially infectious material; contaminated items that would release blood or other potentially infectious material in a liquid or semiliquid state if compressed; items that are caked with dried blood or other potentially infectious materials and are capable of releasing these materials during handling; contaminated sharps; and pathological and microbiological wastes containing blood or other potentially infectious materials
Safety can	An approved container of not more than 5-gallon capacity having a spring-closing spout cover and so designed that it will safely release internal pressure when subjected to fire exposure
Safety Equipment Institute	1901 N Moore Street, Suite 808, Arlington, VA 22209 (703) 525-1695
SARA Title III	Section 302—extremely hazardous substances, 313—toxic chemicals; an amendment to CERCLA called the Superfund Amendment and Reauthorization Act (1986) that also establishes neighborhood right-to-know
Select carcinogen	Any substance that meets one of the following criteria: it is regulated by OSHA as a carcinogen, listed as a known carcinogen by the NTP, listed under Group 1 (carcinogenic to humans) by the International Agency for Research on Cancer Monographs (IARC) or listed in Group 2A or 2B by IARC "reasonably anticipated to be carcinogen" by NTP
Secure landfill	A landfill that is authorized by the EPA or state to receive hazardous waste
Sensitizer	Agents that, with repeated exposure over time, create an allergic reaction at some point in time; reactions may range from minor skin irritation to severe respiratory reactions or even death; most common problem is skin sensitization.
SETA	Setaflash Closed Tester; a type of flash point test
SIC	Standard Industrial Classification
SIR	Standardized Incidence Ratio
SQG	Small Quantity Generator—a generator of 100 to 1000 kg of chemical waste in any given calendar month. For a laboratory, this may be interpreted as the total chemical waste in aggregate per calendar month. SQGs are required to obtain an EPA ID No. before they treat, store, dispose of, or transport hazardous waste; this is referred to as notification and is not considered an application, license, or permit (see also generator).
Solid Waste Disposal Act (1965) , Resource Recovery Act (1970)	Amendments including the Medical Waste Tracking Act
Source individual	Any individual, living or dead, whose blood or other potentially infectious materials may be a source of occupational exposure to an employee. Examples include hospital and clinic patients; clients in institutions for the developmentally disabled; trauma

victims; clients of drug and alcohol treatment facilities; residents of hospices and nursing homes; human remains; and individuals who donate or sell blood or blood components

Stability	Tendency of a chemical to remain in its present state under normal handling and storage conditions (unstable chemicals have a tendency to decompose or undergo other undesirable chemicals changes)
STEL	Short-term exposure limit—maximum concentration to which workers can be exposed for periods up to 15 minutes (see TLV)
Sterility	Changes in male or female reproductive systems resulting in inability to reproduce
Sterilization	A procedure that effectively kills all microorganisms, including bacterial spores
Substance Identification	When calling, you must identify chemical with CAS number or name for assistance (800) 848-6538.
Synergism	The cooperative interaction of two or more chemicals or other phenomena producing a greater total effect than the sum of their individual effect
Systemic Poison	A chemical or other substance that has a toxic effect on the body on one or more of the organs or bodily systems such as lead poisoning
TCC	Tag Closed Cup; type of flash point test
TCLP	Test procedure mandated by the EPA for certain listed chemicals to be landfilled; not applicable to any chemicals used in the clinical laboratory
Teratogen	Materials that may produce deformity of newborns if a significant exposure exists during pregnancy
TLV	Threshold limit value—the airborne concentration of a substance averaged over a normal 8-hour workday or 40-hour workweek (American Conference of Governmental Industrial Hygienists)
TOC	Tag Open Cup—type of flash point test
Toxic Waste	A waste which, by its chemical properties, has the potential to endanger human health or other living organisms by means of acute or chronic adverse effects, including poisoning, mutagenic, teratogenic, or carcinogenic effects
Toxin	Any substance that may cause serious biologic effects when inhaled, ingested, or contacted in small amounts
TSCA	Toxic Substance Control Act (1976) defined more than 44,000 substance as hazardous; requires public notice and hazard assessment of development of any new chemical.
Tuberculosis infection	A condition in which tuberculosis organisms (M tuberculosis, M bovis, or M africanum) are present in the body, but no active disease is evident
Tuberculosis transmission	Spread of tuberculosis organisms from one person to another, usually through the air
TWA	Time Weighted Average; the allowable airborne concentration of a substance for a normal 8-hour day or 40-hour week (see TLV)
UEL	Upper explosive limit
UFL	Upper flammable limit
UN or NA Numbers	United Nations or North American numbers referring to the Emergency Response Guidebook; must be displayed on tank cars, cargo tanks, and portable tanks
UL	Underwriter's Laboratory, 333 Pfingsten Road, Northbrook, IL 60602 (708) 272-1695; recognized independent testing laboratory to which manufacturers submit their products for evaluation of ability to meet safety requirements under intended use
Universal Precautions	A method of infection control in which all human blood and certain human body fluids are treated as if known to be infectious for HIV, HBV, and other bloodborne pathogens

Unstable (Reactive)	Chemical which, in pure state or, as produced or transported, can vigorously undergo autoignition, decomposition, polymerization, can explode or become self-reactive under conditions of shock, pressure, or temperature; reactions of unstable chemicals can result in extremely hazardous conditions.
US Department of Health and Human Services	303 Independence Ave SW, Washington, DC 20201 (202) 619-0257
UV	Ultraviolet
Vacuum Relief Vent	A device to allow air to enter an otherwise closed container to facilitate flow of liquid and prevent collapse due to partial vacuum inside
Vapor Density	A measure of the weight of the vapor compared to the weight of an equal volume of air; vapors such as methane tend to rise quickly and dissipate while others like butane, tend to concentrate in low areas and may present a fire or health hazard (air is given a value of 1)
VP	Vapor pressure
VSD	Virtually safe dose
Water-Reactive	Chemical that reacts with water to release a gas that is either flammable or presents a health hazard
WHMIS	Workplace Hazardous Materials Information System; Canadian Occupational Health and Safety Agency; Workers' Compensation Board of British Columbia, 6951 Westminster Highway, Richmond, BC (800) 972-9972
Work Practice Controls	Controls that reduce the likelihood of exposure by altering the manner in which a task is performed (eg, prohibiting recapping of needles by a two-handed technique)
WWTP	Wastewater Treatment Plant
ZRL	Zero risk level

Mesityl oxide, **78**
Metals, in histology procedures, 67-68
Metanil yellow, **69**
Methacrylate, 94
Methanal. *See* Formaldehyde
Methane, **78**
Methanecarboxylic acid. *See* Acetic acid
Methanoic acid. *See* Formic acid
Methanol, 36, 64, 67, **75**, 93, **94, 194**
Methenyl trichloride. *See* Chloroform
Methyl acetate, **78**
Methyl acrylate, **78**
Methylal, **78**
Methylbenzene. *See* Toluene
Methyl butyl ketone, **78**
Methylene blue, **69**
Methylene chloride, **194**
Methylene violet, **70**
Methyl ethyl ketone, **78**
Methylfluorosulfonate, **145**
Methyl formate, **78**
Methyl green, **69-70**
Methyl isobutyl ketone, **78**
Methyl methacrylate, **78**, 94
Methyl orange, **70, 86**
Methyl propyl ketone, **78**
Microwave oven
  control of health hazards, 105
  federal guidelines concerning, 106
  health hazards, 105
  survey data sheet, **107**
  temperature quality control sheet, **108**
  warning label on, **106**
Mineral oil, 100
Morpholine, **78**
MSDS. *See* Material Safety Data Sheet
Musculoskeletal problems, 23-25
Mycobacteria, 131
Mycobacterium tuberculosis. See
  Tuberculosis program

N

Nanoplast, 94
Naphtha, **78**
B-Naphthylamine, **82**
National Fire Protection Agency (NFPA)
  labeling standards, 71-72
  regulations, **186**
National Pretreatment Program, 99
Nephrotoxin, 63
Neurotoxin, 63, **73**
Neutralization, waste treatment, 202
Neutral red, **70**
NFPA. *See* National Fire Protection
  Agency
NHW. *See* Nonhazardous waste
Nickel, **79**
Nickel carbonyl, **82**
Nickel compounds, **82**
Nickel nitrate, **76**
Nigrosin, **70**
Nile blue, **70**
Nitrate, 36, 193
Nitric acid, 70, **76, 79, 83-85,** 102
Nitrobenzene, **82**

Nitrocellulose, 68, 93
Nitrogen dioxide, **83**
Nitromethane, **78**
Nitrooxantic acid. *See* Picric acid
Nitroparaffins, 35, **85**
Nitrous acid, **79**
Nonhazardous waste (NHW), 184
  examples of, **205**
  incineration of, 199
  liquid, 199
  management of, 199
  minimization of, 199
  recycling of, 199
  segregation of, 199
Notice of Proposed Rulemaking, 7
Notification of Hazardous Waste Activity
  Form (EPA), 201
NRC. *See* Nuclear Regulatory
  Commission
Nuclear fast red, **70**
Nuclear Regulatory Commission (NRC),
  2, 164, **185**

O

Occupational Exposures to Hazardous
  Chemicals Standard, **3,** 4. *See also*
  Laboratory Standard
chemical and other hazards, 87-108
Chemical Hygiene Plan, 49-61
compliance evaluation test, 209
hazardous chemicals, 61-70
labeling requirements, 70-74, **72**
record retention, 8
storage of chemicals, 74-87
Occupational illness/injury
  definition of, 6
  ergonomics, 23-25
  posting information about, 6
  recordkeeping, 6, 8
Occupational Safety and Health Act, **2,** 3
Occupational Safety and Health
  Administration (OSHA), 2, **2-3**
  Bloodborne Pathogen Standard. *See*
    Bloodborne Pathogen Standard
  consultation services, 221-223
  coverage, exceptions, and state
    programs, 5
  deficiencies and problems of, 3-4
  Ergonomic Protection Standard, 24-25
  Formaldehyde Standard. *See*
    Formaldehyde Standard
  General Duty Clause, 5
  Hazard Communication Standard. *See*
    Hazard Communication Standard
  inspection process, 9-10
  laws affecting waste disposal, **185**
  Notice of Proposed Rulemaking, 7
  Occupational Exposures to Hazardous
    Chemicals Standard. *See*
    Occupational Exposures to
    Hazardous Chemicals Standard
  publications by, 219-221
  recordkeeping forms, 6
  record retention guidelines, 8
  reform of legislation, 4

Respiratory Protection Standard. *See*
  Respiratory Protection Standard
standards, 4-5, 220
impact on laboratories, 3
violations of, 9-10
tuberculosis controls, 171, 174
Octane, **78**
Oleic acid, **80**
On-scene incident commander, 90
OPIM. *See* Other potentially infectious
  materials
Organic acids, 77
Organic solvents. *See* Solvents
Organizations, 224-235
OSHA. *See* Occupational Safety and
  Health Administration
Osmium tetroxide, **94**
Other potentially infectious materials
  (OPIM), 197
"Other than serious" violation, 9
Oven. *See* Microwave oven
Oxalic acid, **75, 83, 85**
Oxidizing chemicals, 37, 61
  chemical information about, 36
  frequently used, **37**
  storage of, 76, **76,** 82
  waste, 189
Oxymethylene. *See* Formaldehyde
Ozone, **83**

P

Packaging, of chemical waste, 194
Paraffin, 37, **86**
Paris green, 37
Pathological waste, **196**
PEG-GMA kit, 94
Pelco GMA, 94
Pelco Ultra-low Viscosity, 94
Penalty, for OSHA violations, 9-10
Pentasulfide, **83**
Perchloric acid, **37,** 61, 68, **75-76, 79, 83,
  85,** 93
Permissible exposure limits, 45
Peroxide(s), **85,** 193
Peroxide-forming chemicals, storage of,
  77, **80**
Personal protective equipment (PPE)
  at autopsies, 137
  under Bloodborne Pathogen Standard,
    129, 148-149
  under Chemical Hygiene Plan, 55-56
  for chemical waste handling, 195
  for cryostat use, 142
  under Formaldehyde Standard, 117,
    121-122
  general safety practices, 18
  for infectious waste handling, 195
  information on MSDS, 35
  for radiologic materials handling, 165
  for surgical specimen handling, 139
  in tuberculosis program, 170
  universal precautions, 134-136
Personnel. *See* Employee
Phenoitrinitrate. *See* Picric acid
Phenol, 67, **79, 83**